Fourth
Edition

Nutrition and
Dietetics
Practice and Future Trends

Esther A. Winterfeldt, PhD
Professor Emeritus, Dep[...] of Nutritional Sciences
College of Huma[...] [...]mental Sciences
Oklahom[...] [...]versity
Stillw[...] [...]oma

Margaret L. [...] PhD, RD, LD
Lower Mississippi Delta Nu[...] [...]rvention Research Initiative
Agricult[...] [...]h Service
United States [...] [...]t of Agriculture
Littl[...] [...]kansas

Lea L. Ebro, PhD
Professor Emeritus, Department of Nutritional Sciences
College of Human Environmental Sciences
Oklahoma State University
Stillwater, Oklahoma

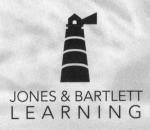

JONES & BARTLETT
LEARNING

World Headquarters
Jones & Bartlett Learning
5 Wall Street
Burlington, MA 01803
978-443-5000
info@jblearning.com
www.jblearning.com

Jones & Bartlett Learning books and products are available through most bookstores and online booksellers. To contact Jones & Bartlett Learning directly, call 800-832-0034, fax 978-443-8000, or visit our website, www.jblearning.com.

Substantial discounts on bulk quantities of Jones & Bartlett Learning publications are available to corporations, professional associations, and other qualified organizations. For details and specific discount information, contact the special sales department at Jones & Bartlett Learning via the above contact information or send an email to specialsales@jblearning.com.

Production Credits

Publisher: William Brottmiller
Managing Editor: Maro Gartside
Editorial Assistant: Agnes Burt
Associate Production Editor: Sara Fowles
Senior Marketing Manager: Andrea DeFronzo
Director of Photo Research and Permissions: Amy Wrynn

V.P., Manufacturing and Inventory Control: Therese Connell
Composition: Lapiz, Inc.
Cover Design: Kristin E. Parker
Cover and Title Page Image: © iStockphoto/Thinkstock
Printing and Binding: Edwards Brothers Malloy
Cover Printing: Edwards Brothers Malloy

Library of Congress Cataloging-in-Publication Data
Winterfeldt, Esther A.
  Nutrition and dietetics : practice and future trends / Esther A. Winterfeldt, Margaret L. Bogle, Lea L. Ebro. —4th ed.
    p. ; cm.
  Rev. ed. of: Dietetics / Esther A. Winterfeldt, Margaret L. Bogle, Lea L. Ebro. 3rd ed. c2011.
  Includes bibliographical references and index.
  ISBN 978-1-4496-7903-3 (pbk.)
  I. Bogle, Margaret L. II. Ebro, Lea L. III. Winterfeldt, Esther A. Dietetics. IV. Title.
  [DNLM: 1. Dietetics. 2. Vocational Guidance. WB 400]
  613.2023—dc23
                                                                                2013001116
6048

Printed in the United States of America
17 16 15 14 13   10 9 8 7 6 5 4 3 2 1

Contents

Introduction

The purpose of this fourth edition of **Nutrition and Dietetics: Practice and Future Trends, Fourth Edition** is to update and present comprehensive information about the profession of dietetics and nutrition and the many career directions and opportunities open to dietitians. This is a profession at the forefront of maintaining healthy lifestyles through prevention and management of nutrition-related diseases and that encourages students of today and tomorrow to take advantage of many unfolding career choices to explore and find professional pathways to a fulfilling and satisfying dietetics career.

This book is about the dietetic profession—what dietitians do, where they practice, and what is required to become a professional dietitian. It is primarily a book for students—those beginning in dietetics, those who are undecided about a career choice, or those who are nearing the completion of their education and training and are exploring additional possibilities. In addition, dietitians or others considering a career change will find information that encourages exploration along new paths of opportunity. Readers will also learn about the historical development of the profession, the Academy of Nutrition and Dietetics, which is the governing body, and the future outlook for dietetics and its practitioners.

Dietitians, through their unique knowledge of both the science and art of nutrition, are the professionals taking the lead in the promotion of nutritional health today. Because of this blend of scientific knowledge and the social and cultural factors that influence what people eat, dietitians are able to use their skills to help individuals in illness and disease prevention as well as those who are healthy and active. Dietitians also interact with professionals of other disciplines that affect nutrition and are able to blend their assorted expertise for the benefit of clients. Their participation in basic research and in integrating new scientific concepts into clinical and public or community nutrition practices adds an invaluable dimension to the dietetics professions.

We have made extensive changes in this fourth edition. They include a newly revised explanation of education and experience requirements; discussion of new and future practice opportunities; updated membership and salary survey data; deletion of some tables and figures and the addition of others; and the results of practice audits and trends in the profession. In addition, all references have been updated and the future explored. Continually expanding opportunities for dietitians are emphasized throughout.

We thank the Academy of Dietetics and Nutrition headquarters staff for timely information and the dietetic experts who contributed to this book through earlier contributions. Their valuable assistance is acknowledged and appreciated.

We hope that students, teachers, advisors, and counselors will find our book informative and motivating in helping make career choices. The authors believe this profession has much to offer and attest that we have enjoyed satisfying and fulfilling careers in this profession. At no time in the past have the opportunities been more appealing for not only a professional dietetics career but also for contributions to families and public service. We hope that many who read this book will be inspired to become dietitians of the 21st century and will help create additional innovative career options.

CHAPTER 1

Introduction to the Profession of Nutrition and Dietetics

"An honorable past lies behind, a developing present is with us, and a promising future lies before us."[1]

OUTLINE

INTRODUCTION

"What is a dietitian?" "What does a dietitian do?"

Recognition of the dietitian as a food and nutrition expert became official in 1917. This, however, was not the actual beginning of the practice of dietetics. The use of diet in the treatment of disease was already an ancient practice even though it was based more on trial and error than on scientific knowledge. Besides physicians, others including home economists, nurses, and cooks were practicing and teaching about good dietary practices, and researchers were uncovering the secrets of nutrients in foods and their health-promoting effect.[2]

Dietetics has been practiced as long as people have been eating. The term derives from *dieto*, meaning diet or food. According to earliest historical evidence, our ancestors were forced to concentrate on simply finding food with little concern about the variety or composition of that food. Today, however, food is plentiful. At least in the developed countries of the world, being able to choose and eat too much from that abundant food supply has become a major problem, resulting in adverse health for many.

Recommendations about eating and food choices have come from biblical admonitions as well as from early physicians and scientists. Physicians in Europe and China, including Hippocrates, formed theories about the relationship between food and the state of a person's health.[3] Many of the early physicians and scientists emphasized adding or eliminating certain foods from the diet according to disease symptoms, although there was not knowledge at that time about nutrients. Until the discovery of the major nutrients in food during the 19th and 20th centuries, a scientific basis for many of the eating recommendations was tenuous at best.

During the 18th century, research by chemists and physicians began to yield information concerning digestion, respiration, and other metabolic functions. The studies were forerunners of later discoveries that identified the elusive substances in foods that were responsible for many of the effects described much earlier in the etiology of disease. Fats, carbohydrates, and amines were known by the mid-1800s, but vitamins and minerals were not discovered until the early 1900s.[4]

One of the most fascinating accounts of the relationship between specific foods and illness is found in Lind's *Treatise of Scurvy* written in 1753.[5] When it was discovered that lemons and limes or their juice would prevent the dreaded scurvy among sailors at sea for long periods of time, it was a lifesaving piece of knowledge. Vitamin C from citrus fruits was later termed the *antiscorbutic* vitamin. Other breakthroughs came when vitamin A was found to be a factor in the prevention of skin lesions and blindness in both animals and people, and when niacin, one of the B-vitamin group, was found to prevent pellagra in humans and black tongue in dogs.[6] There are equally vivid accounts of discoveries of other nutrients.[7]

THE EARLY PRACTICE OF DIETETICS

Cooking Schools

Early cooking schools in the United States, following their emergence in Europe in the early 1800s, led the way toward good dietary practices.[8] One of the first was the New York Cooking Academy founded in 1876, soon followed by schools in Boston and Philadelphia.[9] The schools offered not only cooking instruction but conducted laboratories in chemistry and special classes for the sick.[10] The schools trained many of the men and women who were in charge of food service in hospitals and the Red Cross during World War I.

Hospital Dietetics

Early practitioners in dietetics were in hospitals feeding the sick. Because little was known about people's nutritional needs in either health or illness, food selection was not a major concern. Menus were monotonous and usually featured only a few foods. One account of menus in a New York hospital indicated that mush, molasses, and beer were served for breakfast and supper several days a week. Fruits and vegetables did not appear on menus until later, and then usually only as a garnish.[11]

Florence Nightingale is credited not only with improving nursing of the sick during the Crimean War in the mid-1800s, but also with improving the food supply and sanitary conditions in hospitals.[12]

Clinics

The Frances Stern Clinic in Boston was one of the leading food clinics established in the late 1800s to provide diets for the sick poor. This clinic continues as a leading treatment center and serves as a model for similar clinics throughout the United States.

The Military

Dietitians played important roles during the Civil War and World Wars I and II. During World War I, many served in military hospitals both overseas and in the United States. In World War II during the 1940s, hundreds of dietitians volunteered for active service. Dietitians also worked closely with the Office of the Surgeon General and the Red Cross to help train more individuals in nutrition. Military service and training programs are important professional opportunities for dietitians today.[13]

FOUNDING OF THE AMERICAN DIETETIC ASSOCIATION

The history of the profession of dietetics in the United Stated is also the history of the American Dietetic Association (ADA; now called the Academy of Nutrition and Dietetics) because the two grew together in increasingly important ways. The profession flourished because the association took early steps to oversee both the education and practice of its members. In turn, dietitians supported the association and its activities.

Before the founding of the ADA, persons who worked in food and nutrition programs could join the American Home Economics Association and thus were able to associate and communicate with others of like interests. Dietitians were few in number, and, although they had somewhat similar backgrounds, there was no way to identify persons who were professionally qualified. In 1917, a group of about 100 dietitians met in Cleveland, Ohio, for the purpose of "providing an opportunity for the dietitians of the country to come together and meet with the scientific research workers and to see that the feeding of as many people as possible be placed in the hands of women trained to feed them in the best manner known."[14] Because this was wartime, the government had extensive food conservation programs and used home economists, dietitians, and volunteers to conduct the programs. At the first meeting of the association, officers were elected and a constitution and bylaws were drawn up overnight. Dues were one dollar per year, and there were 39 charter members. Lulu Grace Graves was the first president, and Lenna Frances Cooper was the first vice president.

World War I was, in great part, the impetus that brought early dietitians together to discuss the feeding needs. However, it was also recognized that the services of dietitians in hospitals were rapidly assuming greater importance, both in food service and in treating illness with diet. Researchers were making great strides in nutrition science, and, as more became known about nutrients, maintaining good nutrition and treating certain illnesses with diet became more precise.

The following four areas of practice in dietetics were identified: dieto-therapy, teaching, social welfare, and administration.[15] The vision of the early leaders is evident in that the same four areas of practice exist today, although terminology as well as practice in each area has undergone many changes. The first area, dieto-therapy, or the treatment of disease by diet, was later termed diet therapy, then clinical dietetics, and now is known as medical nutrition therapy or clinical nutrition. Dietitians in the practice of teaching instructed dietetics students, nurses, physicians, and patients. Later called the education section, this group established education standards and specified the experiences needed in an internship to become professionally competent. The social welfare area of practice was later named community nutrition. The administration practice became known as institution administration and later food systems management or management in food and nutrition.

The association continued to grow and by 1927 had 1200 members. The office headquarters were located in Chicago, and the association was legally incorporated in the state of Illinois. The first edition of the *Journal of the American Dietetic Association* was published in 1925, with four issues per year. Early issues of the journal featured subjects similar to those published today, such as hospital food service, personnel issues, and special diets, especially the diabetic diet.

INFLUENTIAL LEADERS

Sarah Tyson Rorer has been credited as the first American dietitian. She was an instructor in one of the early cooking schools and educated both dietitians and physicians in hospital dietetics. Ellen H. Richards was the founder and leader of the home economics movement and so is claimed as one of the early leaders in dietetics. Lulu Graves served as the first president of the ADA and established a training course for hospital dietitians at Cornell University. Lenna Frances Cooper was an early ADA president and director of the School of Home Economics at Battle Creek Health Care Institution in Michigan. Later, she was appointed to the staff of the U.S. surgeon general in Washington, DC. She is commemorated through a lecture presented each year at the annual meeting of the ADA by a current leader in the profession.[16]

Ruth Wheeler prepared the first outline of a training course for student dietitians that established education requirements for dietetics practice. Mary E. Barber, another ADA president, was the director of home economics at Battle Creek and was appointed as a food consultant in 1941 to assist with the problems of feeding 1.5 million soldiers in World War II. She also edited the first official history of the ADA. Mary Schwartz Rose was a leader in nutrition research and nutrition education for the public and established the Department of Nutrition at Columbia University. The Mary Schwartz Rose fellowship for graduate study is awarded yearly in honor of this outstanding scientist and scholar.[17]

Mary P. Huddleston was the editor of the ADA journal from 1927 to 1946. An annual award is presented in her name to the author of the best article published in the previous year's journal. Anna Boller Beach was the first executive secretary of the ADA in 1923, served as president, and was the historian of the association for many years. Lydia J. Roberts was a leading nutritionist at the University of Chicago and the University of Puerto Rico. She initiated nutrition education programs to improve the nutritional status of children in Puerto Rico and was recognized widely for this accomplishment. Mary deGarmo Bryan inspected hospital training courses for dietitians in the 1930s and also developed a training course for directors of school lunch programs.

Scores of other influential leaders led the way in dietetics. Additional information can be found in *Carry the Flame: The History of the American*

Dietetic Association[18] and in the ADA journal. This brief listing highlights those leaders who played key roles in founding the association and thus were pioneers in the profession of dietetics.

DIETETICS AS A PROFESSION

A profession is defined as an area of practice with the following character-istics: specialized knowledge, continuing education, a code of ethics, and a commitment to service for others. Plato first described a profession as "the occupation . . . to which one devotes himself, a calling in which one professes to have acquired some special knowledge used by way of instruc-tion, guidance, or advice to others, or of servicing them in some art."[19] Dietetics, like other professions that fit Plato's description, is organized around these principles in the following ways:

Specialized knowledge. The ADA set standards for education as early as 1919. At least 2 years of college was first recommended, which later became a 4-year requirement or a 2-year course for institutional managers. Courses for the bachelor's degree were specified, and, later, hospital train-ing of 6 months was added to the educational requirement. Subsequent education plans were introduced that continued to specify needed courses. In 1987, standards of education were established, by which dietetics educa-tion focused more on the outcomes of the educational process. The ADA set up a review process that periodically updated educational requirements as the profession grew and matured. Dietitians and employers alike recog-nize the specialized knowledge required to practice in dietetics.

Continuing education. When dietetics was registered as an accredited profession in the 1960s, a requirement of 75 hours of continuing educa-tion each 5 years was initiated. The ADA recognized a wide number of educational events as meeting this requirement and gave credit accord-ingly. Continuing professional education is a well-established function of the ADA through the center for professional education, which offers conferences, annual meeting events, and other opportunities.

A code of ethics. The ADA first developed a code of ethics for its members in 1942.[20] The code was updated an expanded over the years, moving from the *Code of Professional Conduct* to the 2009 *Code of Ethics for the Profession of Dietetics and Process for Consideration of Ethics Issues*. Published jointly by the ADA and the Commission on Dietetic Registration, it provides guid-ance to dietetic practitioners in their professional practice and conduct.[21]

Service to others. The seal of the ADA carried the motto, "*Quam Plurimis Prodesse,*" which means, "benefit as many as possible." Dietitians recognize a professional commitment to help the public attain optimal health and quality of life through the practice of good nutritional habits. The organization reflects this imperative in all areas of practice.

As of January 1, 2012, the name of the association was changed to the Academy of Nutrition and Dietetics.

GROWTH OF THE PROFESSION AND HISTORICAL MILESTONES

Membership

In 1917, the requirements for membership were lenient in order to bring in as many practitioners as possible. Gradually, however, active membership became based on specified education and practical experience. Several categories of membership have been added over the years, and at present, the categories are active, honorary, international, retired, and student members.

Membership in the ADA has risen steadily over the years. The membership grew by about 1000 to 1500 each decade until a growth spurt in the late 1960s, with the addition of about 15,000 members between 1968 and 1978. In 2012, the membership stood at 72,000 of which about 4 percent are men.

Registration and Licensure

In 1969, the association established the system of national professional certification under which the dietitian was designated as a registered dietitian (RD). The title carried legal status and denoted the professional who met the education and experience requirements to practice, in addition to participating in continuing education, thereby maintaining currency of practice. A national testing program was also developed to establish eligibility. Employers soon became familiar with the RD credential and began specifying it as a condition of employment. Today, 75 percent of all dietitians are registered.

Licensure of dietitians occurs in states in which state governments have passed legislation recognizing the profession and awarded state-level legal standing. At present, 46 states have enacted licensure laws for dietitians, many with details of practice allowed, while others promote the title of registered dietitian.[22]

The ADA Foundation

The arm of the association with a tax status identifying it as an educational and scientific nonprofit organization, the American Dietetic Association Foundation (ADAF) solicits and accepts monies donated for scholarships, research, and other designated projects. Several major studies have been funded by the foundation, and programs and lectureships at the annual meeting have been made possible through gifts and donations.

The new title as of 2012 is the Academy of Nutrition and Dietetics Foundation.

Dietetic Technicians and Managers

Managers. The Hospital, Institution, and Educational Food Service Society (HIEFSS) was formed in 1960 as an organization for food service supervisors. It was an independent society but closely tied to the ADA through membership standards as well as financial support. The name was later changed to the Association for Managers of Food Operations (AMFO), and the title for members became food manager. The current name of this association is the Association of Nutrition and Foodservice Professionals (ANFP). Persons completing a voluntary certificate program have the title, certified dietary manager (CDA). Membership stands at over 14,000.

Dietetic technicians. Dietetic technician programs require specific education and training, usually 2 years in a community college program of study. As with the RD, the technician member can also become registered by meeting the specific standards and passing an examination. He or she earns the title dietetic technician registered (DTR).

Several milestones in the history of the DTRs follow[23]:

- *1986.* The American Dietetic Association grandfathered 3618 dietetic technicians into membership.
- *1987.* The first administration of the registration exam for dietetic technicians in nutrition care services and food service systems management was conducted.
- *1987.* The passing standard for the registration examination for dietetic technicians was established.
- *1988.* Continuing education requirements for DTRs were enacted.
- *1990.* First DTR elected to the Commission on Dietetic Registration.

- *1990.* Administration of the first registration examination based on the 1990 role delineation study took place, and new passing standards were developed.
- *1996.* New test specifications for the DTR examination were implemented.
- *2007.* New test specifications for DTR registration examination were implemented.
- *2009.* Pathway III process was implemented to allow didactic program in dietetics graduates to sit for the DTR examination.
- *2011.* Membership stood at 4450.

Legislative Activity

Involvement in legislative activity began when dietitians promoted a bill to grant military rank to dietitians serving in World War I. In the 1940s and 1950s, legislative activity centered around setting standards for employment in the Veterans Administration, passage of the national School Lunch Act, and, in 1946, support of the Maternal and Child Health bill. Signaling even more extensive efforts, the association changed its tax status in the 1960s to permit active lobbying and made its voice heard by establishing an office in Washington, DC, and taking positions on national issues. A political action committee (PAC) was formed in 1980, through which academy members donate funds and recognize legislators who promote legislation on behalf of food and nutrition issues. Each year, the academy identifies key legislative issues for particular attention and activity by the Washington office and members. The current legislative priorities for the academy are discussed later in this text.

Areas of Practice

The practice of dietetics was first structured around four areas in which dietitians were employed. They were: administration, clinical, community, and education. Little was documented about the number of dietitians working in each area until periodic membership surveys were initiated in the early 1980s. As shown in **Table 1-1**, clinical dietetics is the area in which the highest number of dietitians work. Although this initially designated hospital-related dietetics, the clinical dietetics category now includes acute inpatient, ambulatory, and long-term care. The number of dietitians working in food service administration has declined in recent years as more dietitians are now practicing in clinical settings, the community area, and in consultation and private practice.

Table 1-1. Primary Area of Practice by Dietitians (Percent)

Practice Area	1995[1]	2002[2]	2005[3]	2007[4]	2009[5]	2011[6]
Clinical dietetics	45	54	54	55	56	56
Food and nutrition management	26	13	13	12	12	12
Community nutrition	15	11	11	11	11	11
Consultation/ business	7	11	11	11	8	8
Education/ research	7	6	7	6	7	7
Other		5	4	5	6	6

Sources: 1. Bryk, J.A. and T.H. Kornblum. "Report on the 1995 Membership Database of the American Dietetic Association." *J Am Diet Assoc* 97(1997): 197–203.

2. Rogers, D. "Report on the ADA 2002 Dietetics Compensation and Benefits Survey." *J Am Diet Assoc* 103(2003): 243–255.

3. Rogers, D. "Dietetics Salaries on the Rise." *J Am Diet Assoc* 106(2006): 296–305.

4. Rogers, D. "Compensation and Benefits Survey 2007: Above Average Pay Gain Seen for Registered Dietitians" *J Am Diet Assoc* 108(2008): 416–425.

5. American Dietetic Association. Compensation and Benefits Survey of the Dietetics Profession 2009. www.eatright.org. Accessed October 20, 2009.

6. Warde, B. Compensation and Benefits Survey 2011: Moderate Growth in Registered Dietitian and Dietetic Technician Registered, Compensation in the Past 2 Years. 112(2012): 29–40.

Dietetic Practice Groups

Dietetic practice groups (DPGs) are formed by academy members practicing in or having a particular interest in an identified area of practice. DPGs provide a means of networking among group members. The groups elect officers, collect dues, and publish a newsletter or similar communication for its members. From the original 9 groups established in 1978, there are now 28 practice groups.[24] Additional subgroups, or member interest groups (MIGs), have also been formed.

Long-Range Planning

Leaders in dietetics have consistently taken steps to position the profession to meet both present and future needs. This has been achieved through planning groups, task forces, committees, and outside consultants. In 1959, through a study, it was determined that active recruitment, educational opportunities, interaction with other professional groups, and an emphasis on research were needed for continued growth and development of the profession. These goals were expanded in the 1970s with the appointment of a task force and a study commission on dietetics. The study outcome was a report that examined the roles of dietitians and their educational needs for the future. Titled, *The Profession of Dietetics: The Report of the Study Commission on Dietetics*, the report influenced the direction of the association for many years. A second in-depth study in 1984 became a major reference source for long-range planning.[25,26]

Many planning activities that moved the profession forward in significant ways were initiated in the 1980s. The first of a series of long-range planning conferences convened in 1981, with a second in 1984. Invited leaders discussed goals and needs and made far-reaching recommendations. The future was also explored in a strategic planning conference in 1995.[27] The ADA moved decisively toward public outreach and increased involvement in the policy arena, although emphasis on association members and their professional welfare continued.

Further landmark studies examined the education of dietitians, registration and licensure, and advanced practice. In the 1970s, a master plan for education for practice identified trends affecting the demand for dietitians and estimated numbers that would be needed in the future.[28] Role delineation studies included dietetic technicians and described the roles of dietitians and technicians in a variety of settings. These and other studies in the 1990s, including one by the Task Force on Critical Issues: Registration Eligibility and Licensure,[29] continued to show opportunities that enhanced both education and practice and led to continued advances in the profession.

Two task forces in early 2000, the Task Force on the Future Practice and Education and the Phase 2, Future Practice and Education Task Force, initiated broad and comprehensive studies of practice and education.[30]

The board of directors undertakes long-range planning on a regular basis. Using expert consultants and the results of special studies and surveys, the board examines trends impacting dietetic practice to make long-term projections and set goals. The *Strategic Plan of 2011–2012* is the current document outlining the association's goals.

Professional Partnerships

The academy currently maintains liaisons with some 140 allied groups and associations. The formation of these partnerships has advanced mutual efforts and made many programs and activities possible. A long-standing affiliation with the American Public Health Association and the American Diabetes Association has resulted in the development of the diabetic exchange lists and joint publication of the booklet, *Choose Your Foods: Exchange Lists for Diabetes*. Grants from the public health association also allowed the ADA to sponsor workshops on programmed learning. The U.S. Public Health Service sponsors a nutrition section that administers programs critical to health care in the United States. The American Diabetes Association exchanges speakers with the academy at conferences and annual meetings.

The American Hospital Association is another important organization allied with the academy. Hospitals employ many dietitians who contribute to patient care. Hospital-accrediting bodies (e.g., the Joint Commission) include nutrition and food services in their surveys and traditionally with the academy regarding the quality of the services.

The Food and Nutrition Science Alliance (FANSA) was formed in 1992 with the Institute of Food Technology, the American Society for Clinical Nutrition, and the American Society of Nutritional Science. This linkage brought together a combined membership of more than 100,000 who join forces to speak with one voice on food and nutrition issues and to translate scientific information into practical advice for consumers. FANSA is a partnership of seven professional scientific societies whose members have joined forces to speak with one voice on food and nutrition issues.[31]

The American Dietetic Association/Academy of Nutrition and Dietetics has participated in many programs with governmental agencies, including the U.S. Department of Agriculture (USDA), the Department of Health and Human Services (DHHS), the National Institutes of Health, the National Research Council, and the U.S. Congress. Dietitians have served on the Food and Nutrition Board to develop recommended dietary allowances and on the Dietary Guidelines for Americans committee coordinated by the DHHA and USDA.[32]

The International Confederation of Dietetic Associations is composed of 34 national dietetic associations. The American Dietetic Association was an early member of this group. The purposes of the confederation are to achieve integrated communication; promote an enhanced image for the profession; and increase awareness of standards of education, training, and practice in dietetics.

The American Overseas Dietetic Association is affiliated with the academy. The members are academy members living overseas. The members enjoy the same benefits and privileges as other Academy of Nutrition and Dietetics–affiliated groups.

An International Congress of Dietetics is held in a major city every 5 years. The first congress was held in Amsterdam in 1952, with the ADA as one of the founding groups. Organized for the purpose of sharing information, the congress publishes an international bulletin and holds an annual meeting. The 2012 congress was held in Sydney, Australia.

REACHING OUT TO THE PUBLIC

The ADA has initiated many programs over the years directed to the general public. Foremost among the services currently offered by the organization are the academy website, www.eatright.org, and toll-free number, 1-800-877-1600. The website is a source of current information for professionals as well as consumers interested in food and nutrition issues and programs. Employers searching for a dietitian may also use the website to make connections.

Begun as a Dietitian's Week observance in three states, this focus is now a month-long event each March with both local and national emphasis and known as National Nutrition Month.

A dial-a-dietitian program, funded by the Nutrition Foundation, was started in Detroit in 1961. Many states now offer similar services designed to provide information in a timely manner in response to questions from the public.

A training program was initiated in 1982 to prepare selected dietitians to serve as spokespersons for the profession to reach the public with food and nutrition information through the media. More spokespersons, including state media persons, have been added in most major media in the United States. Referred to as the spokesperson network, the program continues to be highly successful at reaching the public with timely and reliable information through television and other media outlets.

Participation in national projects and campaigns is another way the association impacts the public. Over the years, campaigns on women's health, child nutrition, osteoporosis, high blood pressure, and other issues have been the focus of several medical and health-related groups, including the ADA. In 2009, the ADA collaborated with the Alliance for a Healthier Generation to focus on childhood obesity. The alliance is a joint initiative of the American Heart Association and the Academy of Pediatrics, insurance companies, and major media outlets in the initiative on childhood obesity.[33] The national effort to improve the health of the U.S. population is centered in the National Institutes of Health Healthy People 2020 campaign currently under way.[34] The campaign goals are updated every 10 years and include a broad range of U.S. health-related conditions and practices that require attention and improvement. In part because of the participation of professional groups and governmental agencies, this is a program with far-reaching implications for the public.

SUMMARY

The history of the dietetics profession is a rich account of consistent growth, forward-thinking leaders, and the emergence of dietitians as leaders among those concerned with the health and well-being of all citizens. As a profession, dietetics has established standards for practitioner education, a code of ethics, registration and licensure systems, and a tradition of partnership and collaboration with others in allied areas of professional practice to extend outreach and service. The Academy of Nutrition and Dietetics supports its members as they practice in a wide variety of careers, and it also reaches out to the public with timely and reliable information about food and nutrition issues.

DEFINITIONS

Academy of Nutrition and Dietetics. The professional organization for dietitians. Formerly known as the American Dietetic Association.

Dietetic practice group (DPG). An organized group of Academy of Nutrition and Dietetics members with similar interests in an area of practice or a particular subject area.

Dietetic technician. A graduate of an approved dietetic technician program.

Dietitian. A professional who translates the science of food and nutrition to enhance the health and well-being of individuals and groups.

Nutritionist. A professional with academic credentials in nutrition; he or she also may be a registered dietitian.

Registered dietitian (RD). A dietitian who has fulfilled the eligibility requirements of the Commission on Dietetic Registration.

REFERENCES

1. Barber, M.I. *History of the American Dietetic Association (1917–1959).* (Philadelphia: JB Lippincott Co., 1959), p. 3.
2. Corbett, F.R. "The Training of Dietitians for Hospitals." *J Home Ec* 1 (1909): 62.
3. ADA. *A New Look at the Profession of Dietetics. Report of the 1984 Study Commission on Dietetics.* (Chicago: The American Dietetic Association, 1985), p. 29.
4. Todhunter, E.N. "Development of Knowledge in Nutrition. 1. Animal Experiments." *J Am Diet Assoc* 41 (1962): 328–334.
5. Beeuwkes, A.M. "The Prevalence of Scurvy among Voyageurs to America 1493–1600." *J AmDiet Assoc* 24 (1948): 300–303.
6. Goldberger, J. "Pellagra." *J Am Diet Assoc* 4 (1929): 2212–227.
7. McCoy, C.M. "Seven Centuries of Scientific Nutrition." *J Am Diet Assoc* 15 (1939): 648–658.
8. Shircliffe, A. "American Schools of Cookery." *J Am Diet Asoc* 23 (1947): 776–777.
9. See Note 3.
10. Rorer, S.T. "Early Dietetics." *J Am Diet Assoc* 10 (1934): 289–295.
11. Cassell, J. *Carry the Flame: The History of the American Dietetic Association.* (Chicago: The American Dietetic Association, 1990), 4.
12. Cooper, L.F. "Florence Nightingale's Contribution to Dietetics." *J Am Diet Assoc* 39 (1954): 121–127.
13. Mathieu, J. "RDs in the Military." *J Am Diet Assoc* 108, no. 12 (2008): 1984–1987.
14. See Note 11.
15. See Note 3.
16. See Note 11.
17. See Note 11, p. 161.
18. Ibid.
19. See Note 11, p. 5
20. See Note 11, p. 131.
21. American Dietetic Association/Commission on Dietetic Registration. "Code of Ethics for the Profession of Dietetics and Process for Consideration of Ethics Issues." *J Am Diet Assoc* 109, no. 8 (2009): 1461–1467.
22. "State Licensure Information." Academy of Dietetics and Nutrition, Accessed March 11, 2012, www.eatright.org
23. P. Babjak. Personal communication. June 5, 2012.
24. "ADA 2012 Dietetic Practice Groups." Academy of Dietetics and Nutrition, Accessed March 5, 2012, www.eatright.org

25 ADA. *The Profession of Dietetics. The Report of the Study Commission on Dietetics.* (Chicago: The American Dietetic Association, 1972), 2.

26. "The American Dietetic Association Foundation Final Report: 1984. Study Commission on Dietetics: Summary on Recommendations." *J Am Diet Assoc* 84 (1984): 1052–1063.

27. ADA. *ADA Annual Report. 1994–1995.* (Chicago: The American Dietetic Association, 1995), p. 5.

28. Council on Educational Preparation. "Report of the Task Force on Competencies." *J Am Diet Assoc* 73 (1978): 281.

29. Registration Eligibility and Licensure Task Force. *Report of the Critical Issues.* (Chicago: The American Dietetic Association, 1992), p. 10.

30. ADA. *Report of the Phase 2. Future Practice and Education Task Force.* (Chicago: American Dietetic Association, 2008).

31. Food and Nutrition Service Alliance. www.foodprocessding.com/industrylinks. (Accessed April 21, 2012).

32. U.S. Department of Agriculture, U.S. Department of Health and Human Services *Dietary Guidelines for Americans, 2010.* Accessed June 25, 2012, http://health.gov /dietaryguidelines/dga2010/dietaryguidelines2010.pdf

33. "Alliance for a Healthier Generation Expands Efforts to Combat Childhood Obesity with Launch of Landmark Healthcare Initiative." Academy of Dietetics and Nutrition, Accessed August 15, 2009, www.eatright.org

34. Office of Disease Prevention and Health Promotion. U.S. Department of Health and Human Services. "Healthy People, 2020," last modified November 7, 2012, www.healthypeople.gov

CHAPTER 2

The Academy of Nutrition and Dietetics

"Our capacity to influence the public—to *change lives*—is limitless, and it is something we do year-round."[1]

OUTLINE

- Introduction
- The Strategic Plan
- Membership Categories
- Membership Benefits
- Governance of the Academy of Nutrition and Dietetics
  - Board of Directors
  - House of Delegates
  - Accreditation Council for Education in Nutrition and Dietetics
  - Commission on Dietetic Registration
  - Dietetic Practice Groups
- Position Papers
- Dietitian Salaries
- Affiliated Units of the Academy of Nutrition and Dietetics
  - State and District Associations
  - Academy of Nutrition and Dietetics Foundation
  - Washington Office
  - American Overseas Dietetic Association
- Summary
- Definitions
- References

INTRODUCTION

The Academy of Nutrition and Dietetics, formed by a small group of dietitians as the American Dietetic Association (ADA) in 1917, stands as the professional organization of about 72,000 food and nutrition experts (4 percent male and 96 percent female.) In the 95 years since its founding, this organization, which adopted its current name in early 2012, has been the major forum for the networking of dietitians, for research related to food and nutrition, for managerial activities, and for political activities necessary to govern itself.

The original constitution and bylaws of the association have been amended frequently, but the focus of the association has remained constant from the beginning: maintaining a concern for the continuing interests of dietitians and dietetic professionals in their education, practice opportunities, and research for the future. The Academy, as the professional association for practitioners, has long-standing concerns for the protection of the public in areas of nutritional health and disease prevention and the welfare of the practitioner (or individual member). The organization and its leaders of elected members have worked through the years to keep these concerns in focus.

The mission statement of the Academy of Nutrition and Dietetics is, "empowering members to be the nation's food and nutrition leaders."[2] The mission statement sets the agenda of the association and its programs and is described as the association's reason for being. The values that guide the organizational and member behavior are *customer focus, integrity, innovation,* and *social responsibility*.[3] The values are defined as:

Customer focus—meet the needs and exceed the expectations of internal and external customers.
Integrity—act ethically with accountability for lifelong learning and commitment to excellence.
Innovation—embrace change with creativity and strategic thinking.
Social responsibility—make decisions with consideration for inclusivity as well as environmental, economic, and social implications.

The vision of the academy is to "optimize the nation's health through food and nutrition."[4]

THE STRATEGIC PLAN

Through activation of the mission and vision statements along with the identified values and goals, a strategic plan for the academy and its members is in effect. The goals help focus, set priorities, and assign resources. They specify outcomes and represent what needs to be achieved. Three major goals are identified along with 16 strategies to help define how the goals are to be accomplished.[5] The goals are:

1. The public trusts and chooses registered dietitians as food and nutrition experts.
2. The Academy of Nutrition and Dietetics improves the health of Americans.
3. Members and prospective members view the Academy of Nutrition and Dietetics as key to professional success.

In 2008, the ADA adopted a standard logo, replacing a mix of over 100 different visual brands.[6] The logo bears the words, "Eat right."[7]

MEMBERSHIP CATEGORIES

Membership in the academy is available in one of the following categories: active, honorary, retired, student, international, and associate.[8] The associate category is available to members of allied professional groups who are required to hold a minimum of a baccalaureate degree granted by a U.S. regionally accredited college or university or foreign equivalent. The appropriate degree and training, certification, or license in one of 18 food and culinary and health-related professions that meet the qualifications for an associate member are among the requirements.

The largest category of membership is *active*, which generally includes those who hold a baccalaureate degree and have met academic requirements specified by the academy/ADA; an individual with an advanced degree and an emphasis in a closely allied area with dietetics; or a registered dietetic technician (DTR). In addition, any person who has completed a term as president of the association or one who has previously paid dues to obtain life membership may also hold active membership.

The *retired* member category is an option for any member who is at least 62 years of age, either actively employed or no longer employed. *Student* members are those enrolled in an accredited program, a student in a college degree program intending to enter an accredited program, or active members returning to school for a degree in a dietetic-related course of study. *Honorary* membership is awarded to individuals who have made contributions to the field of nutrition or dietetics and are deemed eligible by the board of directors. *International* members are those persons who have completed formal training outside the United States and U.S. territories and have been verified by a country's professional dietetics association or regulatory body.

The rights and privileges of each of the membership categories appear in the bylaws of the Academy. The dues may change from year to year by action of the house of delegates. Dues differ for each category, with a portion of the national dues offsetting the cost of the Journal of the Academy of Nutrition and Dietetics and a rebate returned to the state affiliate associations for each member of the state. In addition, the national dietetic practice groups (DPGs) charge for membership in their groups and provide newsletters and other educational materials for members in the specific practice area.

MEMBERSHIP BENEFITS

Membership in the academy benefits the individual and collective members in many ways.[9] These may be summarized under the following categories:

- Information sources
- Publications and electronic newsletters
- Career resources
- Practice resources
- Social networking
- Educational opportunities
- Policy initiatives and advocacy
- Science and quality
- Networking and promotions
- Promotional resources
- Additional benefits

GOVERNANCE OF THE ACADEMY OF NUTRITION AND DIETETICS

The organizational structure of the ADA/Academy of Nutrition and Dietetics changed over time; however, governance has been through members who were either elected, appointed, or volunteered from the membership at large. Those elected each year are the officers serving on the board of directors, delegates to the house of delegates (HOD) by states, members of the Commission on Dietetic Registration, and members of the Accreditation Council for Education in Nutrition and Dietetics (ACEND). Members of the foundation board are appointed, and membership in dietetic practice groups (DPGs) is by member choice. A chief executive officer (CEO) is employed by the board to oversee and manage a paid staff at the headquarters in Chicago. Under the leadership of the CEO, the staff members form partnerships with the various volunteer groups, forming teams to accomplish the variety of tasks necessary to keep the organization functional and to implement the strategic plan. The board of directors (BOD) and the HOD function as a voice for members.

Board of Directors

The BOD is composed of 18 members: president, president-elect, past president, treasurer, treasurer-elect, three directors at large, six HOD directors, two public members, the foundation chair, and the CEO, who is nonvoting. The BOD governs the organization through the following activities:

- Sets and monitors strategic direction
- Oversees fiscal planning
- Provides leadership for professional initiatives
- Selects, supports, and assesses the CEO and conducts an annual performance appraisal
- Appoints persons to represent the association
- Establishes guidelines and policies for appeals, publications, awards, and honors
- Administers and enforces the professional code of ethics
- Exercises powers and performs lawful acts under the Illinois Not-for-Profit Corporation Act

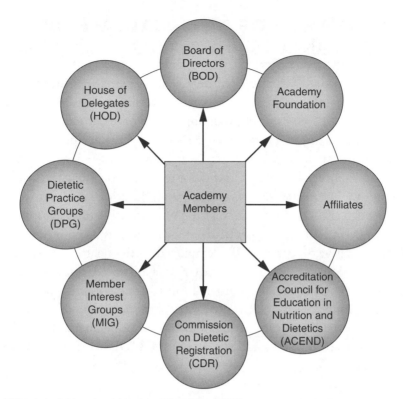

The HOD includes (total number of delegates = 106 as of June 1, 2012):

- *6 Affiliate Delegates* are elected by members of the 53 affiliate dietetic associations.
- *28 Dietetic Practice Group Delegates* are elected or appointed by DPG membership and represent the specific DPG from which they are elected/appointed.
- *6 At-Large Delegates*: one delegate representing ACEND (appointed by ACEND), one delegate representing CDR (appointed by CDR), one delegate representing student members (elected by the Student Advisory Committee), one delegate representing DTRs (elected nationally), one delegate representing retired members (elected by HOD), and one delegate representing members under 30 years of age (elected by HOD).
- *6 HOD Directors* comprise the House Leadership Team (HLT), including the Speaker, Speaker-elect, and immediate Past-Speaker, elected by the membership. They are members of the Academy Board of Directors (BOD).

HOD Vision Statement: The House of Delegates, as the voice of members, governs the profession and develops policy on major professional issues.

To govern the profession of dietetics, the HOD engages in the following activities:

- Monitors and evaluates trends affecting the profession,
- Monitors member issues and mega issues, and the resulting actions,
- Approves standards of education and standards of practice,
- Reviews, debates, and approves professional standards,
- Establishes the size and structure of the House,
- Adopts and revises with the Commission on Dietetic Registration (CDR) a code of ethics for dietetics practitioners, disciplinary procedures for unethical conduct, and reinstatement conditions,
- Makes recommendations on standards, qualifications, and other issues related to credentialing to the Commission on Dietetic Registration,
- Makes recommendations on accreditation, approval and related issues to the Accreditation Council for Education in Nutrition and Dietetics (ACEND),
- Provides direction for quality management in dietetics practice,
- Identifies and develops position statements,
- Provides oversight to Academy Bylaws and,
- Assists with recruitment and retention efforts related to Academy membership, plus leadership development.

FIGURE 2-1. Academy of Nutrition and Dietetics Organization Units.

Source: Used with permission from the Academy of Nutrition and Dietetics, 2013.

House of Delegates

The house of delegates (HOD) is composed of 110 affiliate delegates representing the 53 affiliate dietetic associations who are elected by the affiliate members. In addition, there are 18 professional issues delegates representing the DPGs who are elected by the general ADA membership. Ten at-large delegates are also in the house, representing groups as follows: one from ACEND, one delegate representing the Commission on Dietetic Registration, two dietetic technician delegates, one representing student members, one representing retired members, one representing members under 30 years of age, and three delegates from the total membership. Finally, six HOD directors who comprise the house leadership team and are elected by the BOD.

The HOD provides a forum for membership and professional issues and establishes and maintains professional standards of the membership. Core roles of the HOD include adopting and maintaining a code of ethics in conjunction with the CDR, developing position statements and other professional papers, establishing qualifications and dues of members, and the formula for dues payment to affiliate organizations. The HOD also identifies and prioritizes trends and recommends policy and strategic direction for the academy. The HOD has the authority to establish committees and rules and policies of organization and governance, including its own composition and size.

Both the BOD and the HOD represent academy members and govern the academy. As a comparison, the BOD is likened to the executive branch of the U.S. government and the HOD to the legislative branch. Both groups work together closely to promote the interests of the members and further the profession.

Accreditation Council for Education in Nutrition and Dietetics

The Accreditation Council for Education in Nutrition and Dietetics (ACEND) establishes and enforces standards for the educational preparation of dietetics professionals and recognized dietetics education programs that meet the standards. The ACEND administers and has authority for all actions that apply to accreditation of entry-level education programs that include standard setting, fees, finances, and administration. There are 12 members on the council. At least half of the members represent each program type (dietetic technician, didactic, coordinated, and dietetic internship). The council includes 1 representative of other constituents, a dietetic student, and 2 representatives of the public.

Commission on Dietetic Registration

The mission of the Commission on Dietetic Registration (CDR) is to protect the public through credentialing and assessment procedures that assure the competence of registered dietitians and dietetic technicians, registered and specialists.

The CDR sets the standards for certification and recertification and enforces the code of ethics of the association. The commission issues credentials to those individuals who meet the standards. Dietitians thus attain the registered dietitian (RD) designation, and dietetic technicians the DTR. Specialists receive the certified specialist title.

Dietetic Practice Groups

Dietetic practice groups (DPGs) are professional interest groups within the academy framework. The 28 active groups show the diversity of the practice areas in which dietitians work (**Table 2-1**). Each group networks to serves its members, charges fees to support its activities, and maintains communication with its members by various means. The groups also sponsor educational sessions at the annual meeting. The requirements to join a DPG are academy membership or registration status and payment of dues. A member may belong to as many groups as desired.

Formation of new groups occurs after interest groups become large enough to seek official status. A petition is submitted with no fewer than 500 signatures indicating interest, individuals willing to serve as officers, and a budget. Aside from maintaining a minimum of 300 members, other uniform requirements include publication of a newsletter at least quarterly for its members, maintaining governing documents, conducting an annual meeting of its members, and maintaining a balanced budget. DPGs offer networking opportunities with professionals with similar interests and provide significant opportunities for leadership responsibilities both within the DPG and the academy.

Table 2-1. Dietetic Practice Groups 2013–2014

2013–2014 Dietetic Practice Groups (DPGs)	Description
Behavioral Health Nutrition (BHN) DPG	BHN members are the most valued source of food and nutrition services for persons with addictions, eating disorders, intellectual and developmental disabilities and mental illness.
Clinical Nutrition Management (CNM) DPG	Managers who direct clinical nutrition programs across the continuum of care.
Diabetes Care and Education (DCE) DPG	Members involved in patient and professional education, plus research for the management and prevention of diabetes.
Dietetic Technicians in Practice (DTP) DPG	Members are advocates for dietetic technicians, registered, as dietetics practitioners in providing quality client care.
Dietetics in Health Care Communities (DHCC) DPG	Practitioners providing nutrition consultation to acute and long-term-care facilities, home care companies, healthcare agencies, corrections, and the foodservice industry.
Dietitians in Business and Communications (DBC) DPG	Food and nutrition practitioners who work for or consult with corporations, businesses, and organizations, or who are self-employed or business owners.
Dietitians in Integrative and Functional Medicine (DIFM) DPG	Food and nutrition practitioners that promote the integration of conventional nutrition practices with evidenced-based alternatives including functional and integrative medicine and nutrition genomics.
Dietitians in Nutrition Support (DNS) DPG	Dietitians who integrate science and practice of enteral and parenteral nutrition to provide nutrition support therapy to individuals (adults, pediatrics, inpatients, outpatients, home care, transplantation and complex gastrointestinal disorders).
Food and Culinary Professionals (FCP) DPG	Members who love food, as well as promoting food and culinary skills. Specialty groups include supermarket, restaurant and retail food service and food safety.
Healthy Aging (HA)DPG	Practitioners leading the future of dietetics in the aging community by promoting independence and well being through health promotion, chronic disease management strategies and public policy advocacy.

(continues)

Table 2-1. Dietetic Practice Groups 2013–2014 *(continued)*

2013–2014 Dietetic Practice Groups (DPGs)	Description
Hunger and Environmental Nutrition (HEN) DPG	Members who lead the future in sustainable and accessible food and water systems through education, research, and action.
Management in Food and Nutrition Systems (MFNS) DPG	Food and nutrition care managers generally employed in health care institutions, universities, corrections, and other facilities.
Medical Nutrition Practice Group (MNPG) DPG	Practitioners who practice a wide range of medical nutrition therapy across the continuum of care in a variety of settings. Now includes DPG #29 Infectious Disease Nutrition (IDN) as a subunit.
Nutrition Education for the Public (NEP) DPG	Practitioners involved in the design, implementation, and evaluation of nutrition education programs for target populations.
Nutrition Educators of Health Professionals (NEHP) DPG	Members involved in nutrition education of health care professionals.
Nutrition Entrepreneurs (NE) DPG	Members shape the future of dietetics practice by pursuing innovative and creative ways of providing nutrition products and services to consumers, industry, media, and business.
Oncology Nutrition (ON) DPG	Nutrition practitioners involved in the care of patients with cancer, cancer prevention, and research.
Pediatric Nutrition (PNPG) DPG	Practitioners who lead in promoting optimal nutritional health through education, research and service of infants, children and adolescents.
Public Health/Community Nutrition (PHCNPG) DPG	Nutrition practitioners who work in public health nutrition and community nutrition settings.
Renal Dietitians (RPG) DPG	Practitioners who provide medical nutrition services to chronic kidney disease patients in dialysis facilities, clinics, hospitals, university settings, and private practice.
Research (RDPG) DPG	Members who conduct research in various areas to promote practice standards, health policy, and disease prevention.
School Nutrition Services (SNS) DPG	School foodservice directors, nutrition educators, and corporate dietitians working in the delivery of food service and nutrition education to children.

(continues)

Table 2-1. Dietetic Practice Groups 2013–2014 *(continued)*

Sports, Cardiovascular, and Wellness Nutrition (SCAN) DPG	Nutrition practitioners with expertise and skills in promoting the role of nutrition in physical performance, cardiovascular health, wellness, disordered eating and eating disorders.
Vegetarian Nutrition (VN) DPG	Nutrition practitioners who serve as the leading authority on evidence-based vegetarian nutrition (plant based diets) for health professionals and the public.
Weight Management (WM) DPG	Practitioners who work in the prevention and treatment of overweight and obesity throughout the life cycle.
Women's Health (WH) DPG	Practitioners addressing women's nutrition care issues during the reproductive period through menopause.

Source: Printed with permission: Academy of Nutrition and Dietetics.

A practice group may also develop subunits or groups of members within the DPG based on a practice area or issue of interest to the members of the group, thus creating an even smaller group of dietitians with closely allied interests. Currently, 28 subspecialty areas exist within the main DPGs.

In addition, member interest groups (MIGs) have been formed whereby specific population groups can share mutual interests.

POSITION PAPERS

A position paper represents a consensus of viewpoints and professional interests and is used in many ways such as in media contacts, in drafting legislation and testifying before governmental groups, and for communication with the public. A nutrition position paper is described as a statement of the association's stance on an issue that affects the nutritional status of the public; it is derived from pertinent facts and data and is germane to the academy's mission, vision, philosophy, and values. Position papers are periodically updated or deleted, and others added by the HOD. Copies of current position papers are available from the academy headquarters office or at www.eatright.org.

DIETITIAN SALARIES

The salary levels of dietitians and dietetic technicians have risen over the years, with certain practice areas commanding higher salaries. These changes reflect the increasingly important roles played by dietitians and dietetic technicians. In 1938, it was reported that hospital dietitians, on the average, earned an annual salary in the range of $1090 to $7000. At that time, benefits such as room, board, and laundry were often supplied by the employer in addition to a salary. In positions other than those offered by hospitals, the salaries ranged from $1200 to $4000 per year. In 1946, the average salary was reported to be $3000—not a significant improvement.[10]

In 1981, the ADA initiated the first survey of members that reported salaries along with other data regarding employment. At that time, the average yearly salary was $16,000, although the study did not equate all salaries with full-time practice and the actual full-time salaries were probably higher.[11] The median yearly salary for dietitians in all areas of practice from 2002 through 2011 is shown in **Table 2-2**. In 2011, the median salary for dietitians was $57,990.

Table 2-2. Median Income for Registered Dietitians by Area of Practice

Practice Area	2002[a]	2005[b]	2007[c]	2009[d]	2011[e]
Clinical	42,825	47,923	51,668	55,390	56,056
Food and nutrition management	55,000	60,008	64,002	67,995	70,990
Community nutrition	43,200	44,803	48,006	52,000	51,120
Consultation/ business	60,000	53,768	60,008	69,992	65,000
Education/ research	54,800	60,216	66,061	65,000	64,000
All areas	45,800	49,500	53,000	56,700	57,990

Sources: a. Rogers, D. "Report on the American Dietetic Association Dietetics Compensation and Benefits Survey." *J Am Diet Assoc* 103 (2003): 243–265.

b. Rogers, D. "Dietetics Salaries on the Rise." *J Am Diet Assoc* 106 (2006): 296–305.

c. Rogers, D. "Compensation and Benefits Survey 2007: Above-Average Pay Gain Seen for Registered Dietitians." *J Am Diet Assoc* 108 (2008): 446–425.

d. American Dietetic Association. "Compensation and Benefits Survey of the Dietetics Profession 2009," accessed at www.eatright.org.

e. Ward, B. "Compensation and Benefits Survey 2011: Moderate Growth in Registered Dietitian and Dietetic Technician, Registered, Compensation in the Past 2 Years." *J Acad Nutr Diet* 2012 (1): 29–40.

When comparing salaries by areas of practice in dietetics, it is apparent that dietitians in food and nutrition management have the highest incomes while those earning the least are in community nutrition practice. Several factors account for differences in compensation, including years in a position, education level, job responsibilities, number of persons supervised, budget responsibility, and location.[12]

The median wage for the registered dietitian technician was $30,659 in 2002, $34,000 in 2005, $36,000 in 2007, $39,000 in 2009 and $40,000 in 2011.[13]

AFFILIATED UNITS OF THE ACADEMY OF NUTRITION AND DIETETICS

State and District Associations

Each of the 50 states and Puerto Rico are affiliates of the academy and are organized with state and district associations. Membership in the academy determines the membership in state affiliates because states generally charge no membership fees and instead receive rebates from the academy according to the number of members. A member of the academy is automatically a member of a state affiliate.

The state organizations for the most are parallel to the national organization. Each state elects its delegates to represent its members in the HOD. The number of district organizations is determined by the states as well as how they fit into the state organization. The district groups provide educational and informational programs for the grassroots members. Most states have one or two meetings per year that provide continuing education opportunities for the members. Delegates from the state take state and/or member issues to the HOD for all members to have input into the functioning of the academy.

Academy of Nutrition and Dietetics Foundation

The Academy of Nutrition and Dietetics Foundation is a nonprofit arm of the academy that solicits and receives monies to benefit the academy, with a large percentage of the monies going to provide scholarships for both undergraduate and graduate students and for member research projects. The foundation fosters alignment with corporate sponsors and conducts member campaigns for fund-raising. The foundation also provides services for the public in various ways.

More than 900 students have been awarded scholarships since 2007, totaling nearly $1.4 million. The Evidence Analysis Library, a resource offered through the foundation, is a member-accessible online reference library housing relevant nutritional research on important dietetic practice questions. The service is also available through a subscription service to others.[14]

Washington Office

In 1986, the ADA began staffing an office in Washington, DC, in order to have a presence in the capital and to further the legislative efforts of the profession. This allows the association to be in touch with legislative issues as they are being considered and as they occur. Although these legislative and lobbying efforts required a tax status change by the association when they were first initiated, the benefits accrue to individual members directly and to consumers and the public indirectly.

The staff of the Washington office and academy members work with legislators and government agencies to introduce and promote bills that further the interests of the profession and its members. An example is the passage of the Medical Nutrition Therapy Act, which resulted from a sustained effort on the part of ADA staff together with legislators over several years.

American Overseas Dietetic Association

Dietitians who have met all requirements for membership in the academy are eligible for membership in the overseas association. They may join dietetic practice groups and enjoy all the same benefits of membership as they would in the United States.

SUMMARY

The Academy of Nutrition and Dietetics is the professional organization serving and promoting the interests of its members. The programs and initiatives administered by the academy are for the benefit of the members and the public. The academy is governed by elected and appointed volunteer members of boards, commissions, and committees, all of whom perform specific functions according to the bylaws of the academy. Important as the functions that the academy provides for members are, it is recognized as the authoritative voice to the public with guidance regarding food and nutrition issues. The active promotion of policy that enhances the health and well-being of all individuals is accomplished through activities by members and by the Washington legislative office.

DEFINITIONS

Bylaws. Authoritative rules governing an association or group.

Chief executive officer (CEO). A person employed by the association to direct the headquarters office operations and implement the programs and fiscal affairs of the association. May also serve as an official spokesperson for the academy on direction of the board of directors.

Governance. Activities involved in conducting the affairs of an organization.

Strategic plan. Plans and strategies that shape the overall activities and functions of an organization.

REFERENCES

1. Escott-Stump, S.A. "President's Page." *Acad Nutr Diet J* no. 3 (2012): 352.
2. "ADA's Strategic Plan Roadmap". www.eatright.org (Accessed January 5,2012).
3. See Note 2.
4. See Note 2.
5. See Note 2.
6. Switt, J.T. "The American Dietetic Association's New Look." *J Am Diet Assoc* 108 (2008): 932–933.
7. See note 6.
8. Escott-Stump, S.A. Communication by email to members. June 21, 2011.
9. Lipscomb, R. "2012 Academy Member Benefits Update." *Acad Nutr Diet J* 112 (2012): 468–475.
10. Cassell, J. *Carry the Flame: The History of the American Dietetic Association.* (Chicago: The American Dietetic Association, 1990).
11. Baldyga, W.W. "Results from the 1981 Census of the American Dietetic Association." *J Am Diet Assoc* 83 (1983): 343–348.
12. Ward, B. "Compensation and Benefits Survey 2011: Moderate Growth in Registered Dietitian and Dietetic Technician, Registered, Compensation in the Past 2 Years." *Acad Nutr Diet J* 1 (2012): 29–40.
13. See Note 12.
14. Academy of Nutrition and Dietetics website, accessed November 5, 2012, www.eatright.org.

CHAPTER 3

Educational Preparation in Dietetics

"As a profession, the one thing that we can predict is that the greatest change in our practice will be the change in knowledge and how we integrate new science into our daily practice."[1]

INTRODUCTION

Education is the key to dietetic practice and to the future of the profession. As with all professions, a specialized body of knowledge is required of individuals who practice in any area of dietetics. Because of the importance of education to the profession, the early leaders in dietetics set standards for education of dietitians. The standards have been revised at intervals as the practice evolved and the needs of those being served changed.

UNDERGRADUATE EDUCATION

The educational preparation of dietitians begins in the undergraduate degree program. Study for the baccalaureate degree is based in the biological, physical, and social sciences and includes both a theoretical and applied course of study. The college or university offering a degree program plans a curriculum that meets both the educational standards of the Academy of Nutrition and Dietetics and the university requirements, including courses for general education. A baccalaureate degree from an accredited college or university, combined with supervised practice integrated into the degree program or an internship following the degree is necessary to complete all education requirements. A program that offers the practical experience component concurrent with the degree is termed a coordinated program (CP). A curriculum that meets the academy education standards is referred to as a didactic program in dietetics (DPD). The dietetic technician (DT) similarly follows a course of study in a 2-year college or institute that includes or is followed by supervised practice experience.

PROGRAM REQUIREMENTS

The Accreditation Council for Education in Nutrition and Dietetics (ACEND) sets the standards by which dietitians are educated. The standards have been issued in various forms since 1924 and have undergone many changes in both concept and format. For instance, early emphasis was on the specific courses a student was required to take during a degree program. Now, the standards are based on the outcomes expected from the education experience, and education program directors translate the expected outcomes into courses and course content.[2] The ACEND further specifies how a degree program is to be structured, including the goals and philosophy of the program, the students, the curriculum, the program resources, and the evaluation of the program.

The program standards for both the didactic and the experience components are the following[3,4]:

1. *Program eligibility for accreditation.* This includes program characteristics and finances, Title IV compliance, and requirements as consortia.
2. *Program planning and outcomes assessment.* The program has clearly defined its mission, goals, objectives, and assessment methods. Ongoing program improvement is to be documented.
3. *Curriculum and student learning objectives.* The curriculum plan, length, learning activities, and learning assessments are specified.
4. *Program staff and resources.* Responsibilities of the program director, the faculty and preceptors, continuing professional development, program resources, and supervised practice facilities are included in this standard.
5. *Students.* Plans for student progression and professionalism, student complaints, information provided to prospective students and the public, as well as policies and procedures followed in the program are to be included in this standard.

The ACEND evaluates each educational program through a site visit based on an extensive self-study program prepared by the program director and staff. The purpose of the site visit by registered dietitians designated by the academy is to assist the program in continued assessment that ensures qualified, competent program graduates who pass the registration examination and are prepared to practice. A program may be accredited for a period of 1–10 years. Periodic reports are submitted by the program director to the academy indicating that a program continues to provide education that meets the standards.

A list of all accredited programs is available from a college or university or from the academy website.

DIETETICS EDUCATION REQUIREMENTS

The route to becoming a registered dietitian is based on the study of a wide variety of topics focusing on food, nutrition, and management. These areas are supported by the biological, physiological, behavioral, social, and communication sciences. A combination of academic preparation including a baccalaureate degree and a supervised practice component completes the preparation for entry-level practice.

Foundation Knowledge and Competencies

The current educational standards were issued in 2012 after a revision of earlier standards. Input was obtained from faculty, administrators, students, practitioners, and employers, resulting in their development. The learning outcomes from the use of these standards are outlined under five areas representing foundation knowledge for DPD programs and competencies for dietetic internships. The five areas follow.

1. *Scientific and evidence base of practice.* Integration of scientific information and research into practice.
2. *Professional practice expectations.* Beliefs, values, attitudes, and behaviors for the professional dietitian level of practice.
3. *Clinical and customer services.* Development and delivery of information, products, and services to individuals, groups, and populations.
4. *Practice management and use of resources.* Strategic application of principles of management and systems in the provision of services to individuals and organizations.
5. *Support knowledge.* Knowledge underlying the requirements as specified.

DIETETICS EDUCATION PROGRAMS

Didactic Program in Dietetics

The didactic, or classwork, portion of the dietetics educational requirements is completed during the degree program (either undergraduate or
graduate). Following degree conferral, the student completes a supervised practice program or internship. The traditional didactic program
in dietetics (DPD) is a 4-year undergraduate bachelor of science degree.
Many of the courses required in the DPD combine classroom and laboratory work, especially courses in food production, clinical nutrition, and
science courses such as chemistry and microbiology.

During the later part of the program, usually the senior year, the student applies to one or more dietetic internships through a computerized
matching program. Notification is given in April or November about a
match or acceptance to the student's program of choice. After completion
of the supervised portion of the program, the student may take the registration examination.

Coordinated Program in Dietetics

In the coordinated program (CP) in dietetics, the didactic portion of
a program and supervised practice are completed during the course
of study toward the degree, either undergraduate or graduate. The
student graduating from this program is thus prepared for entry-level
practice upon completion of the degree. In most universities, students
enter the CP for their junior and senior years. The program is sometimes
referred to as "two by two," meaning the first 2 years are general study
and may be at a community or junior college and the last 2 include
the integrated courses leading to the degree. Some programs may be
longer than the traditional 4 years depending on the specific program
requirements.

A university designates the criteria for admission to the CP. The selection criteria commonly include grade point average, writing skill, work
experience, letters of recommendation, and sometimes, an interview.
A minimum of 1200 hours of supervised practice is required in the CP.
The CP is intense in terms of time requirements and experiences but can
reduce the time needed to prepare for practice. On completion of the
degree, the student is eligible to take the registration examination.

Dietetic Technician Program

The dietetic technician (DT) program is similar to the coordinated program in that both didactic knowledge and skills and supervised practice (a minimum of 450 hours) are required in the program. The requirements are specified and programs are accredited by the ACEND. Graduates of the program are eligible to take the registration examination for DTRs and for entry-level practice. Many of these programs are offered in 2-year colleges or in technical schools.

TRENDS IN DIETETICS EDUCATION

Summit on Dietetics Practice, Credentialing, and Education

The education of the dietitian focuses on the present and future roles professionals will fulfill. The traditional roles continue to expand as environmental, demographic, business, and health trends create new opportunities for practice.[5] In the 2011 Future Connections Summit on Dietetics Practice, Credentialing, and Education,[6] several suggestions were presented that directly impact the education of dietitians. Among these were the following:

- RDs will want to become "adaptable generalists," developing a career that will probably include numerous jobs with continued reeducation as needed.
- Continuing education coupled with lifelong learning will enable keeping pace with advancements within health care and technology. Alternatives to traditional classroom-based education will need to emerge.
- Education needs to be career oriented versus job oriented with preparation for ongoing critical thinking skills.
- A learner-centered approach to education will be needed rather than one that is more traditional, i.e., teacher-oriented.
- Undergraduate education will need to emphasize writing skills, analytic skills, and ability to learn independently to develop attitudes essential in a caring profession that contribute to the society of which they are a part.

Council on Future Practice Visioning Report 2011

The Council on Future Practice was established in 2009 by the academy in response to recommendations of the Phase 2 Future Practice and Education

Task Force to address specific recommendations of the Phase 2 Task Force and monitor progress of the academy, the CDR, and the ACEND toward meeting these recommendations.[7] The first charge of the council was to conduct a visioning process to identify/define future practice roles and the broad knowledge and skills needed for these roles. As a result of this visioning process, three sets of materials were developed initially: The *Dietetics Career Development Guide and Related Definitions; Definitions for Focused Areas of Dietetic Practice, Specialist and Advanced Practice*; and visioning process results.[8] The *Dietetics Career Development Guide* shows the progression of the practitioner through at least five stages of perceptions of the job, changing skill levels, and decision making as the individual progresses from novice to the expert stage. Conceptually, this guide is based on the Dreyfus model of skill acquisition.[9] For each stage, a definition, rationale, and criteria for practice (education, experience, and demonstrated examples) are given for RDs, DTRs, specialists, and advanced practice dietitians.

Envisioned practice roles for DTRs and RDs (entry-level generalists, health promotion/disease prevention specialists, public policy makers, clinical healthcare specialists, education specialists, researchers, food production workers, and service managers and food industry workers) for 2020 were defined. Likewise, future roles for specialists (neonatal nutritionists, genomics specialists, nutrition informatics specialists, chronic disease managers, community/public health nutritionists, etc.) and for advanced practice RDs (health promoters/disease prevention specialists, researchers, clinical healthcare workers, systems specialists, and services managers, etc.) were delineated. This report presents the most complete and detailed information that the academy has made available to practitioners in guiding their careers for the future practice in dietetics for many nontraditional as well as enhanced traditional roles.

Distance Education

Distance education is the means by which many colleges and universities now offer courses and degree programs. With the increased use of technology by both students and practitioners, such offerings are often attractive to part-time students, older returning students, and those who reside away from the university setting. Three universities currently offer the DPD, and one offers the CP by distance.[10]

A graduate eight-university consortium that allows students to take online courses toward a degree in any of the eight universities is described in the Summit Conference of 2011.[11] A dietetics curriculum is among several graduate degrees that are offered. Distance education is also increasingly used in dietetic internships, and, currently, 16 programs offer all or some of the required learning by distance.

Continuing education opportunities for professionals are increasingly offered by distance through webinars, teleconferences, teleseminars, and various social networking means. The annual public policy workshop was offered only in Washington, DC, until 2011, when it was first offered by distance. Many dietetic practice groups regularly communicate through online linkages such as blogs, LinkedIn, Facebook, and Twitter.

A new concept in providing patient care is described as "telehealth" provided through "telepractice."[12] Telehealth is defined as active or passive interaction with patients to support long-distance clinical health care, patient and professional health-related education, public health, and health administration. When, for instance, medical nutrition therapy is offered via a webcam, it is described as telepractice or "the interactive use of electronic information and telecommunication technologies to engage in the diagnosis, education, and treatment of patients as clients at a remote location through means such as teleconferencing."[13] There are legal considerations and other limitations that apply in the use of all such technology, and many are discussed in some detail in a 2010 *Journal of The American Dietetic Association.*[14]

A survey in 2011 of over 3000 ADA members showed that members are adopting and using electronic technology in their practice. The average positive response was 3.77 on a 5.0 scale with about one-fourth of the respondents being highly experienced. In decision making, the average response was 4.3 of 5.0.[15]

SUPERVISED PRACTICE IN DIETETICS: DIETETICS INTERNSHIP

Preprofessional or supervised practice is an essential step toward becoming an RD or DTR. For the DPD student, the dietetic internship follows the degree. Supervised practice takes place in the work setting where students learn to apply their knowledge and skills under the direction of an RD preceptor. Successful completion of a supervised practice program establishes eligibility for an individual to take the registration examination and to apply for active membership in the academy. Competency in dietetics practice is the goal of supervised practice. Competency is regarded as the ability to carry out tasks within certain expected standards or parameters.

Supervised practice programs are based on the standards of education and the competencies for entry-level practice. All supervised programs are provided through an accredited program and must offer a minimum of 1200 hours of experience for the dietitian and 450 hours for the dietetic technician. A current listing of all programs is available on the academy website (www.eatright.org).

All programs follow the same standards; however, there is flexibility in the way programs meet the standards through the kinds of experiences offered. Although the ACEND accredits educational programs, it does not mandate the kinds of experiences or the amount of time in each area of practice. Each program sets the curriculum and experiences that meet the goals of the program and the needs of the student.

Program experiences are structured around the following three key areas of activity in dietetics: clinical nutrition, food service management, and community dietetics. Programs that do not offer all the experiences in one institution will arrange with others in the community to provide them.

Supervised experience is offered through the dietetic internship, the coordinated program, and the dietetic technician program. A new avenue, the individualized supervised practice pathway (ISPP), became available in 2011.[16] The ISPP is available for graduates who were verified by their university as meeting undergraduate requirements but were not matched during the internship application process. The program does allow individuals with a doctoral degree and dietitians from overseas to apply without a verification statement.

The following questions are often asked when students apply to supervised practice programs:

What do students need to know before applying?
What are the characteristics of successful applicants?
What else is important to know?

These questions will be answered next.

What do students need to know before applying? Students should know that a period of supervised experience is required to establish eligibility to become an RD or DT, and that acceptance into a program is competitive. The application process should begin early in the senior year in order to assemble all required materials by graduation and, if required by the program or desired by the student, to visit one or more programs. Students applying for a dietetic internship usually will participate in national computer matching, and this information may be obtained from the program director or from the academy office.

What are the characteristics of successful applicants? Generally, applicants with a grade point average of 3.0 or above in food, nutrition, and management courses and better than average grades in biological and physical science courses will be considered first. Approximately 1 year of work experience or dietetics-related volunteer or paid experience will increase the chances of being accepted.

What else is important to know? In addition to good grades and having work experience, applicants are encouraged to investigate programs early to identify the specific admission criteria and to apply to one or more programs. Successful applicants often apply to as many as three programs. If the program offers graduate credit during the supervised experience, the student will also need to apply to graduate school and complete the graduate record examination (GRE). In addition, applicants are encouraged to be flexible and be willing to relocate if necessary.

ADVANCED-LEVEL EDUCATION

Advanced-level education may be described as continuing education, postprofessional education, or graduate education. More baccalaureate students are pursuing a graduate degree; more employers are requiring an advanced degree, training, or advanced credentials; and more disciplines are becoming specialized, thus requiring advanced-level education. Graduate education is formal study beyond a baccalaureate degree that leads to an advanced degree, i.e., the master's or doctoral degree. Graduate study involves concentrated study in a specific academic area. Some universities offer or require graduate study concurrently with the dietetic internship.

Among the important purposes of advanced education are opportunities for individuals to explore new ideas and to gain a higher level of knowledge and understanding required to recognize and fully discharge personal, social, and professional responsibilities. Practical benefits also accrue, including networking with other advanced practitioners and specialists, the possibility of career advancement, and financial gain.

Types of Programs

The master of science (MS) degree usually requires 1–2 years of full-time study and may be longer depending on the major area of study, the research undertaken, and whether the student attends school full- or part-time. In some universities, the MS is offered with the option of a thesis or a creative component and additional course work instead of the thesis.

The doctor of philosophy (PhD) degree requires at least 3 years of full-time study. The PhD or the EdD (doctor of education) may be offered. Original research is required for either degree, the type depending on the field of study. Currently, some universities are requiring two to three publications in peer-reviewed journals and/or a dissertation as a requirement for graduation. The doctoral degree is considered the terminal degree, although it may be followed by postdoctoral academic work.

Healthcare team members for other allied health disciplines have been offering a practice doctorate for advanced level practice as an alternative to the PhD. Currently this is occurring in pharmacy, occupational therapy, physical therapy, and nursing.[17] It seems appropriate that there be a dietetic practice doctorate for advanced practice RDs on the team as well. This was first proposed in 1993 but was not well accepted.[18] However this is now happening in at least one university in the United States and is being discussed in others.[19] In addition, many universities are offering traditional doctoral degrees in clinical nutrition management, nutrition genomics, nutrition informatics, etc., all of which are referenced in the future roles of dietetics practice. See a listing of advanced degree offerings in the United States at www.eatright.org.

Benefits of Advanced Study

The benefits of an advanced degree include the development of intellectual skills, including the ability to master complex information, to problem solve, and to explore new ideas. Career benefits include the development of advanced practice skills, the in-depth exploration of subjects in one's area of practice or another focus of practice, and the acquisition of new perspectives. Dietitians often pursue graduate study for career advancement or preparation for a career change. Dietitians who are prepared to perform in multiskilled or cross-trained positions will usually rely on graduate education to increase their knowledge and practice skills.

The types of positions dietitians assume as they progress up the career development guide are usually those with increasing responsibility and autonomy, and they require managerial and leadership skills. In addition, competition for jobs may increase the demand for an advanced degree. New and expanding career options and the job market in general affect demand and availability of a person prepared to enter the new job markets and, in turn, influence dietitians in their education choices. Graduate education provides an opportunity to develop expertise that allows dietitians to assume leadership roles.

In the 2011 Dietetics Compensation and Benefits Survey, it was reported that almost 50 percent of RDs hold an advanced degree. Among DTRs, 35 percent hold a bachelor's degree or higher.[20]

The financial advantages of an advanced degree for RDs are shown in **Table 3-1**. Attaining an advanced degree increases, on the average, the yearly wages of registered dietitians by $5000 (MS) and $20,000 (PhD). State licensure and specialty certification affect salaries and are often equated with advanced study. Dietitians working in practice areas that often require an advanced degree, such as food and nutrition management and education and research, earn the highest salaries.

For DTRs, the median wage was $40,000, an increase of 2.6% since 2009. The factors affecting these salaries are the same as for the RD—education, experience, responsibility, and location. The DTRs in food and nutrition management generally earn the highest salaries.

Table 3-1. Median Yearly Income of Registered Dietitians by Education Level

	2009[a]	2011[b]
All RDs	$57,000	$58,000
Master's degree	60,000	60,000
Doctoral degree	83,000	75,000
Bachelor's degree	54,000	55,000

a. American Dietetic Association. "Compensation and Benefits Survey of the Dietetics Profession 2009," Accessed www.eatright.org

b. Ward, B. "Compensation and Benefits Survey 2011: Moderate Growth in Registered Dietitian and Dietetic Technician, Registered, Compensation in the Past 2 Years." *Acad Nutr Diet J* 112 (2012): 29–40.

A further justification for the RD to pursue graduate study is for continuing education credit to maintain registration status. State licensure regulations may mandate an advanced degree and continuing education as well.

Active membership in the academy is available to an individual holding a master's or doctoral degree in one of the following areas: dietetics, food and nutrition, nutrition science, food science, or food service systems management. The degree must be from a regionally accredited college or university.

Gaining research skills and understanding research articles and reports is a further benefit of graduate study. All dietitians apply research in their practice and need to demonstrate the ability to interpret current research and basic statistics. However, designing and participating in formal research usually occur at the graduate level.

The Graduate Program Experience

Information about graduate programs offering degrees in dietetics or closely related subject areas is available in the academy directory of programs or from universities. Prospective students will find it helpful to talk with faculty and to request college catalogs and departmental information before applying. No two programs are alike, and the best fit between the student and a program will be important once the student is admitted. Universities that give students an active role in departmental activities and that give individual time and attention in a mentoring and supportive atmosphere will greatly enhance the graduate experience. The faculty, departmental research, and the availability of financial aid through graduate assistantships should also be explored. Assistantships not only provide financial aid but give the student teaching, research, and/or administrative experiences according to assignments.

Research Experience

The selection of a research study by the student with an advisor is based on the area of interest, the need as determined by a literature search, and the feasibility of the study (based on cost, time involvement, and availability of equipment and/or subjects). Ongoing departmental research by faculty can provide a way for the student to assume a part of the research for his or her thesis.

The process of investigating a problem, reviewing the literature to support the need for the study, planning and implementing the study, collecting and analyzing data, and writing a clear and well-developed document that is accepted by a graduate faculty committee is a significant effort. The research experience requires initiative, critical thinking, problem solving, and ethical procedures. These are aspects of professional functions that are vital to success in life, as well as a career. The successful completion of a research study often launches a student into publishing the results and into further research, thus making an important contribution to scholarship.

Further Opportunities

The leadership in the academy and the ACEND are concerned and have been taking steps to overcome the disparity between the number of DPD graduates and the availability of dietetic internships for all who wish an internship experience.[21] Among the steps being taken is the recent notice that DPD students who have completed the degree are now allowed to sit for the DTR examination and work as a dietetic technician. The new ISPP program will also allow more graduates to attain internship experiences. The CDR approved funding the Academy of Nutrition and Dietetics Foundation to provide support for the establishment of advanced practice residency programs across the spectrum of dietetics practice.[22] Several pilot initiatives for residency programs are under way with the goal of enhancing advanced practice and to provide a pathway for registered dietitians as delineated by the Guidelines for ACEND-Accredited Advanced Practice Residencies (1.0) were released in 2012, and indications are that additional guidelines will be published after a series of pilot residencies are completed.[23]

Program directors who advise students and students themselves need to have other options in mind when an internship appointment is not obtained. Some will plan to gain more working experience and then reapply. A suggested alternative is to consider an advanced degree; after attaining it, membership in the academy is available, and teaching and research opportunities may follow. Some students gain additional training or complete course work to enter allied health areas such as nursing, physician assistance, or physical therapy. Employment areas that in most cases do not require the RD credential might also be considered. Examples of these are pharmaceutical companies, journalism and communications, the hospitality and management industries, athletic training spas and centers, tourism, retirement homes, cooperative extension, and school food service.

SUMMARY

Dietetics education has evolved over time but has always been based on preparing the student for professional practice. The academy designates the educational standards that are followed by all dietetics programs, thus ensuring competent practitioners. With a background of academic knowledge and practical skills, dietitians and dietetic technicians are prepared for a wide variety of careers as described in other chapters in this text.

Almost half of practicing dietitians today hold or are working toward a graduate degree. There are benefits in doing so—among them are the attainment of research competence, continuing education for personal and professional growth, and career enhancement. If the trend continues, ever-larger numbers of dietitians will seek an advanced degree and will thereby bring expertise to bear on practical problems in food, nutrition, and health. The outcome will be a healthy and informed public and heightened recognition of the dietitian as the expert in food and nutrition.

DEFINITIONS

Accreditation. The process whereby a private nongovernmental agency or association grants public recognition to an institution or an individual who meets necessary qualifications and periodic evaluation.

Advanced practice. The practitioner who demonstrates a high level of skills, knowledge, and behaviors. The advanced practice individual exhibits a set of characteristics that include leadership and vision and demonstrated effectiveness in planning, evaluating, and communicating targeted outcomes.

Coordinated program. A degree program combining didactic and experiential learning.

Dietetics. The integration, application, and communication of principles derived from food; nutrition; and social, business, and basic sciences to achieve and maintain optimal nutrition status of individuals through the development, provision, and management of effective food and nutrition services in a variety of settings.

Preceptor. A person who guides, mentors, and evaluates a student during the supervised practice experience.

Specialist. A practitioner who demonstrates a minimum of the proficient level of knowledge, skills, and experience in a focus area of dietetics practice by the attainment of a credential.

Supervised practice. Learning experiences associated with activities in selected situations that enable the student to apply knowledge, develop skills, and develop professionally.

REFERENCES

1. Parks, S.D., M.R. Schiller, and J. Bryk. "President's Page: Investment in our Future—The Role of Science and Scholarship in Developing Knowledge for Dietetics Practice." *J Am Diet Assoc* 949 (1994): 1159–1161.
2. Commission on Accreditation for Dietetics Education. "Eligibility Requirements and Accreditation Standards for Didactic Programs in Dietetics," Academy of Dietetics and Nutrition. Accessed February 24, 2012, www.eatright.org
3. Commission on Accreditation for Dietetics Education. "CADE Accreditation Standards for Didactic Programs in Dietetics (DPD),"Academy of Dietetics and Nutrition. Accessed April 3, 2012, www.eatright.org
4. Commission on Accreditation for Dietetics Education. "CADE Accreditation Standards for Dietetic Internship Programs (DI)," Academy of Dietetics and Nutrition. Accessed April 3, 2012, www.eatright.org
5. Council on Future Practice. *Council on Future Practice Visioning Report.* (Chicago: The American/Dietetic Association, 2011).
6. Boyce, B. "2011 Future Connections Summit on Dietetics Practice, Credentialing, and Education: Summary of Presentations on Shaping the Future of the Dietetics Profession." *J Am Diet Assoc* 2011 (211): 1591–1599.
7. Report of the Phase 2 Future Practice and Education Task force. (Chicago: The American Dietetic Association, 2008).
8. See Note 5.
9. Dreyfus, H. L., and S. E. Dreyfus. *Mind Over Machine.* (New York: The Free Press, 1986).
10. Personal communication. Academy of Dietetics and Nutrition. Accessed April 3, 2012, www.eatright.org
11. See Note 6.
12. Raun, L. "Telehealth." *Ventures* 2010, no. 3 (XXVI): 15.
13. See Note 12.
14. Aase, S. "Toward E-Professionalism: Thinking Through the Implications of Navigating the Digital World." *J Am Diet Assn* 110, no. 10 (2010): 1442–1449.

15. Ayres, F.J. "2011 Nutrition Informatics Member Survey." *J Am Diet Assn* 112, no. 3 (2012): 360–367.
16. Wilson, A. "New Supervised Practice Pathway Offers Additional Options to Dietetics Graduates." *ADA Times* 9, no. 1 (2011, Autumn): 18–19.
17. Touger-Decker, R. "Advanced-Level Practice Degree Options: Practice Doctorates in Dietetics." *J Am Diet Assoc* 104 (2004): 1456–1458.
18. Christie, B.W., and M.A. Kite. "Educational Empowerment of the Clinical Dietitian (A Proposed Practice Doctorate Curriculum)." *J Am Diet Assoc* 93 (1993): 173–176.
19. Skipper, A., and N.M. Lewis. "Clinical Registered Dietitians, Employers, and Educators Are Interested in Advanced Practice Education and Professional Doctorate Degrees in Clinical Nutrition." *J Am Diet Assoc* 106 (2006): 2062–2066.
20. Ward, B. "Compensation and Benefits Survey 2011: Moderate Growth in Registered Dietitian and Dietetic Technician, Registered, Compensation in the Past 2 Years." *J Acad Nutr Diet* 112 (2012): 29–40.
21. Wilson, A. "Creating Our Competition: Why the Dietetic Internship Shortage is as Important to Your Future as It Is to the Practitioners of Tomorrow." *ADA Times* (2010, Winter 2010): 12–15.
22. See Note 21.
23. Accreditation Council for Education in Nutrition and Dietetics. "Guidelines for ACEND-Accredited Advanced-Practice Residencies," Academy of Nutrition and Dietetics. Accessed April 1, 2012, www.eatright.org

CHAPTER 4

Credentialing of Dietetic Practitioners

"Experts at curing diseases are inferior to specialists who warn against disease. Experts in the use of medicines are inferior to those who recommend proper diet."[1]

OUTLINE

INTRODUCTION

The term *dietitian* is one that evolved over time. Early practitioners were called dietologists, dietists, and dietotherapists.[2] Before the American Dietetic Association (ADA) was formed, a dietitian was described as "a person who specializes in the knowledge of food and can meet the demands of the medical profession for diet therapy."[3] This adequately described the professional for many decades.

The developing science of food and nutrition formed the basis for the organization of a group of practicing professionals. One of the earliest concerns of this group was the overwhelming amount of food faddism and fallacies found among the general public and even among other professionals. It was difficult, if not impossible, for the public to determine who was a credible source of information and to separate fact from fiction between the many medical and health claims for specific foods and procedures.

This early concern for protection of the public by disseminating the knowledge of dietitians has continued to the present time. Not only did it lead to the national organization of dietitians that could promote the professionals as having expertise in "diet-therapy, teaching, social welfare, and administration,"[4] but it served as the impetus to begin thinking about credentialing of practitioners.

A concern raised at the second annual meeting of the ADA in 1918 was the "need to distinguish between dietitians with a college degree and special training in some scientific work and the ones with lesser training."[5]

This was perhaps the first formal reference to dietetic credentialing. The 1926 president of the association, Florence Smith, urged that the group establish professional standards for dietitians and that state or national registration could be the answer. In 1929, a study of national registration was initiated, and the following definition of a dietitian was adopted: "'Any person who is qualified for membership in The American Dietetic Association is by virtue of uniform basic training and required experience, entitled to be designated as a dietitian."[6] In the 1950s, the association appointed a committee to formally study state licensing of dietitians. The issue of specialties in practice also surfaced with the suggestion that membership should be expanded to include others who were well qualified in the many specialties embraced within the definition of dietetics.[7] However, it was in the late 1990s that education and membership requirements were differentiated to accommodate practitioners with similar basic preparation but in specialized areas of practice.

The differences between a generalist and a specialist surfaced and were thoroughly debated. A generalist was defined as a dietitian who could perform in all areas of practice, such as a single dietitian in a small hospital, or one who could move from one practice area to another. A specialist was a dietitian wanting to restrict his or her practice in one area, such as clinical or food service. The generalist role was advanced by the following themes:

1. All dietitians are the same.
2. Dietitians can move from one area of practice to another (food service to public health, for example) without additional training.
3. Greater external recognition of the term *dietitian* was established.

By contrast, the specialized role was driven by the following themes:

1. The explosion of knowledge and technology required each dietitian to know more and more about less and less.
2. There was a need to differentiate among dietitians with varying skills and knowledge, advanced education, and experience gained on the job.
3. Part-time employment opportunities emerged.
4. New, innovative practice areas developed, such as school food service, nursing home consultation, enteral and parenteral nutrition techniques, and nutrition support.

DEVELOPMENT OF CREDENTIALING

In the 1960s, a committee was established to study licensure, registration, and certification. Registration was the credentialing process chosen at that time by the ADA house of delegates and the ADA membership. An amendment to the constitution was approved for the *Final Revised Proposal for Professional Registration* in 1969. A committee, later to become known as the Commission on Dietetic Registration (CDR), then began the implementation of a certification process for members. The title for those ADA members who chose to become certified was registered dietitian (RD). A detailed account of the implementation and a review of the first 5 years of professional registration were published in the *Journal of the American Dietetic Association* in 1974.[8]

The professional registration system adopted by the association differed significantly from other health professional certification systems at that time in that candidates had to pass a national examination, and RDs had to document evidence of continuing education in each 5-year period to renew registration. Thus registration was designed as a voluntary process to ensure competency of dietitians through the qualifications required to take the registration examination, passing the examination, and formal continuing education. All of this was evidence of the concern of the profession for the health, safety, and welfare of the public by encouraging high standards of performance by dietetic practitioners as stated in the amendment to the constitution.[9]

Ninety percent of the membership was registered by the end of the 1970s, with the majority grandfathered in during the period before establishment of the examination. Credentialing of the dietetic technician and various dietetic specialists followed with qualifications developed by the Commission on Dietetic Registration.

COMMISSION ON DIETETIC REGISTRATION

The Commission on Dietetic Registration (CDR) is the agency responsible for maintaining the registration process for the former American Dietetic Association, now known as the Academy of Nutrition and Dietetics (AND; referred to as the Academy). This group develops, revises, and administers the examination for registration; sets the standards for certification and recertification; establishes the Code of Ethics for the Profession of Dietetics jointly with the Academy; and issues credentials to individuals who meet these standards for competency to practice in the dietetics profession. The mission statement of CDR is, "Protecting the nutritional health and welfare of the public through dietetics certification."[10]

Registered Dietitian

The examination to become an RD is administered online (prior to this advancement it was offered in written form at designated sites twice a year), and individual applicants can schedule a time to take it throughout the year. The examination is also available in other countries from organizations with which the academy has reciprocity. Currently those are Dietitians in Canada, the Dutch Association of Dietitians, the Philippine

Professional Regulation Commission, the Irish Nutrition and Dietetic Institute, and the Health Professions Council of United Kingdom.

The eligibility requirements for individuals to take the examination to become a registered dietitian are the following:

- Complete the minimum of a baccalaureate degree from a U.S. regionally accredited college or university or foreign equivalent
- Meet current minimum academic requirements (didactic program in dietetics) accredited by the Accreditation Council for Education in Nutrition and Dietetics (ACEND) of the academy. Additional information (including a directory of accredited programs) and updates on academic and supervised practice programs can be found on the ACEND website at www.eatright.org
- Complete supervised practice pathways (ISPPs) through ACEND-accredited programs to accommodate the increased demand of students.[11] This text and the ACEND website at www.eatright.org provide accurate and current information as to the type and length of supervised practice requirements.

After passing the examination and being credentialed by the CDR, registered dietitians are required to comply with CDR recertification requirements, the code of ethics for the profession of dietetics, and the standards of practice.

Dietetic Technician, Registered

The dietetic technician, registered (DTR) is a critical member of the dietetics team and becomes even more important as the practice of dietetics in every area becomes more complicated and time consuming. Dietetic technicians are trained in food and nutrition and are an integral part of health care, food service, and other dietetics and healthcare teams. In small, rural hospitals, the DTR is sometimes the only trained dietetics practitioner addressing all aspects of care available full time. In this situation, the DTR works under the supervision of an RD via established protocols to implement the nutrition care process based on state regulations. At present, only Maine has state licensure procedures for the dietetic technician. The Scope of Dietetic Practice Framework guidelines for licensure address supervision, entry-level, and advanced practice for DTRs.[12]

The role of the dietetic technician must be recognized, strengthened, and supported. An increase in the number of DTRs is vital to sustain expansion of practice areas for dietitians and achieve the future vision for the profession.

The small number of DTRs and dietetic technician educational programs place this segment of our profession at risk for continued existence. Steps must be taken to ensure a sufficient number of DTRs to meet demand and achieve the future vision of the dietetics team who need DTRs as viable team members to succeed.

In addition, a realistic and workable career ladder within the dietetics profession must be created and implemented as quickly as possible. The opportunity for advancement, moving from dietetic technician to registered dietitian to advanced practitioner, must become a reality. A functional career ladder will strengthen the dietetics profession as we seek to enhance the recognition, authority, autonomy, prestige, income, and satisfaction of dietetics team members and their customers.

It is well known that DTRs work in nontraditional or emerging areas of practice with more diverse possibilities for the future. After years of practice, DTRs also may work with RDs in advanced-level practice areas such as renal dietetics. The use of the standards of practice and standards of professional performance for dietetic technicians, registered partially addresses this issue of advanced practice for DTRs.[13] The DTR works under the direction of the RD in the provision of clinical nutrition services or medical nutrition therapy. The DTR practices in food service management, community programs, and in evolving settings and organizational structures. Depending on the complexity of the organization, the DTR may or may not work under the supervision of the RD.

The opportunities for employment keep expanding for the DTR, especially in areas where supply of RDs cannot meet the demand. More and more employers, especially in the healthcare arena, are requiring that an individual be credentialed as a DTR in order to practice in their facilities. Some current unique opportunities are:

- Supervising food safety and sanitation in a variety of public and private venues
- Assisting individuals and groups in wellness and fitness centers to know how food relates to fitness
- Managing and directing food service employees in assisted living and retirement centers
- Assisting the RD in collecting data from patients or participants in research studies (in hospitals, clinics, and community research centers)

The *Final Report of the Phase 2 Future Practice and Education Task Force* provides much detail of innovative educational experiences and unique roles and employment for DTRs both now and in the future.[14]

The DTR of today will extend the scope of practice for the RD in the future and will allow the RDs to delegate responsibilities, enabling them to practice at specialty and advanced levels. However, for this to happen, the RD must understand the role and appropriate responsibilities of the DTR, which in many instances will increase visibility and credibility of the dietetic professional team and will benefit clients, facilities, the RD, and the profession of dietetics. Last but not least, the dietetics profession and the academy must promote the value of DTR educational programs and the dietetic technician as a creditable member of the team for practice in tomorrow's world.

New DTR Registration Eligibility Pathway

For the past several years, the CDR and others have noted the decline in the number of DTRs. This decline has been complicated by the lack of educational programs for DTRs in many states; many employers have been unable to hire DTRs, which has increased the unavailability of DTRs in many parts of the United States. The CDR has supported the role of the dietetic technician and believes that a new pathway will address both of these issues. This decision is consistent with the CDR's public protection mission in that it provides a credential for the numerous noncredentialed didactic program in dietetics (DPD) graduates currently employed in dietetic technician positions. Once credentialed as DTRs, these individuals will be required to comply with the CDR recertification requirements and the standards of practice and the code of ethics for the profession of dietetics.[15] The CDR also believes that this alternative registration eligibility option will provide a dietetics career ladder, increase the availability and visibility of DTRs throughout the country, and ultimately enhance the value of the DTR credential.[16] The *Dietetics Career Development Guide* uses the Dreyfus model of skill acquisition to show how practitioners can attain increasing levels of knowledge and skills throughout a career.[17]

Therefore, at its April 2009 meeting, the CDR established a new registration eligibility pathway for dietetic technicians. Effective June 1, 2009, individuals who have completed both a baccalaureate degree and a DPD will be able to take the registration examination for dietetic technicians without meeting additional academic or supervised practice requirements. This decision also provides for the numerous non-credentialed DPD graduates currently employed in dietetic technician positions to become credentialed. Once credentialed, these individuals will be required to comply with CDR recertification requirements and the code of ethics for the profession of dietetics and the standards of practice. The CDR also believes that this alternative registration eligibility option will increase the availability and visibility of DTRs throughout the country, ultimately enhancing the value of the DTR credential.

Effective June 1, 2009, the three pathways to establish eligibility to take the registration examinations for dietetic technicians are:

1. *Pathway A.* Completion of an associate's degree granted by a U.S. regionally accredited college or university with the Accreditation Council for Education in Nutrition and Dietetics (ACEND) Accredited Dietetic Technician Program.
2. *Pathway B.* Completion of a baccalaureate degree granted by a U.S. regionally accredited college or university, or foreign equivalent, completion of an ACEND-accredited DPD, and completion of an ACEND-accredited dietetic technician supervised practice.[18]
3. *New pathway.* Completion of a baccalaureate degree granted by a U.S. regionally accredited college or university, or foreign equivalent, and completion of an ACEND-accredited DPD or an ACEND-accredited Coordinated Program in Dietetics (CP).

For security reasons, all candidates must be processed through the Credential Registration and Maintenance System (CRMS) for eligibility to take the examination issued by their DPD program director. All candidates must complete an electronic application available on the CDR's website at http://cdrnet.org/vault/2459/web/files/DTRPathway3.pdf; and the DTRE Mis-Use Form at: http://cdrnet.org/vault/2459/web/files /DTRE%20%20Mis-Use%20%20-%20%20Updated%204-09.pdf. After passing the registration examination for dietetic technicians and being credentialed by the CDR, dietetic technicians, registered, are required to comply with CDR recertification requirements, the code of ethics for the profession of dietetics, and the standards of practice.

The following are additional Academy of Nutrition and Dietetics' webpages of importance to individuals preparing for certification as dietetic technicians:

Examination Candidate Information and Study Resources:
Computer-based testing FAQ:
> http://www.cdrnet.org/certifications/rddtr/cbtfaq.htm

Study Guide for the Registration Examination for Dietetic Technicians, 5th edition:
> http://www.eatright.org/cps/rde/xchg/ada/hs.xsl/shop_9603_ENU_HTML.htm

Check It Out—Becoming a Dietetic Technician Registered:
> http://www.eatright.org/students/education/becomeregistered.aspx

Specialist Certification

In 1986, the concept of specialized practice in dietetics was approved by the house of delegates. The ADA defined a specialty as an advanced level of practice that responds to a defined area of need and requires demonstrated competency exceeding that for entry-level practice. Specialty areas must have a substantial and verifiable knowledge base, an identified dimension of advanced practice, and a reasonably sized pool of practitioners. Three areas of practice were selected for initial certification: pediatric nutrition, renal nutrition, and metabolic nutrition care.[19] The first specialty areas were chartered in 1994. The metabolic nutrition care specialty was later discontinued.

In 2010 the Academy added a focus area of dietetics practice to the *specialist* definition, indicating that specialists responded to a practice that requires focused knowledge, skills, and experience. The new definition of a specialist is, "a practitioner who demonstrates additional knowledge, skills and experience in a focus area of dietetics practice by the attainment of a credential."[20] New criteria were established for the specialist, which include education and experience requirements as well as the successful completion of the CDR examination in the focus area. Currently specialists are credentialed in the following areas:

Gerontological nutrition
Sports dietetics
Pediatric nutrition
Renal nutrition
Oncology nutrition

An additional area of recognition was developed in 1993 for those practicing at advanced levels in any area of dietetics.[21] The Fellow of the American Dietetic Association (FADA) was available until 2003 for those having an advanced degree, 8 years of practice, plus other documented professional achievements.[22] This recognition was discontinued because of limited participation of members of the association; however, research and discussion within the academy continues to attempt to address the issue of career ladders and levels of practice, including advanced practice.[23–26] Future roles and definitions for RDs, DTRs, specialists, and advanced practice were delineated in 2011 by the Council on Future Practice.[27]

Certificates of Training

Currently the CDR offers three certificates of training in weight management. Responding to the epidemic of obesity and the need for registered dietitians to become more involved in the efforts to prevent and treat obesity, the CDR provides workshops across the United States resulting in certificates in childhood and adolescent weight management; adult weight management, and a level 2 certificate in adult weight management. The certificate programs are designed to develop practitioners of comprehensive weight management care for adults, children, and adolescents. The certificates are available for ADA members, RDs, and DTRs. Training for the certificates includes:

- State-of-the-art information and skills shared by leading practitioners
- Hands-on experience with cases and exercises
- Reference and other resource materials
- A range of 32 to 50 continuing professional education units (CPEUs) depending on the individual certificates

This training and the subsequent certificates have become very useful and popular with dietetic professionals returning to the workplace, working in private practice, and to registered dietitians in general. There is no reissue of the certificates, but certificate holders are encouraged to participate in retraining as needed. Additional information can be found at the CDR website (www.cdrnet.org).

Recertification of the RD and DTR

In 2001, the CDR implemented a new process for continued certification termed the professional development portfolio (PDP).[28] To maintain registered status, RDs and DTRs must participate in the CDR's mandatory

PDP recertification system and remit the annual registration maintenance fee. Using this plan, the individual RD and DTR assumes the responsibility for learning, professional development, and career direction. The PDP requires each practitioner to first engage in self-reflection, followed by assessment and goal setting. This process is followed by the development of a 5-year plan that reflects a critical analysis of goals and the steps to be taken to maintain professional competency.[29-32] The academy's standards of professional practice and the CDR's professional development portfolio mutually assure competence of the dietetics practitioner.

As greater numbers of registered dietitians retire, maintaining competence and adhering to the code of ethics for the profession will present challenges, especially for those maintaining RD status. A recent article by Dahl and Nye discusses this issue, which could be viewed as relevant to all practitioners, in detail.[33]

Participation in continuing professional education activities is essential for lifelong development to maintain and improve knowledge and skills for competent dietetics practice. RDs and DTRs must report CPEUs using the portfolio recertification system. The process by which the required 75 CPEUs are accumulated is also determined by the CDR, which specifies the educational activities that qualify to be used as CPEUs. Beginning with the 5-year recertification starting in 2012 and ending in 2017, RDs and DTRs are required to complete 1 CPEU in ethics (Learning Need Code 1050).[34]

To remain registered, an RD is required to pay yearly dues and engage in 75 hours of continuing education over a 5-year period. A DTR pays dues and must accrue 50 hours in a 5-year period. In the past, RDs and DTRs could not report more than 75 and 50 CPEUs, respectively, for the 5-year period. Beginning in 2011 they were able to accrue rollover CPEUs as long as they meet specific requirements. The details can be found at the CDR website (www.cdrnet.org) under the Professional Development Resource Center.

Recertification of Specialists

The specialty board certification is a practice credential (just as RD and DTR are) that represents to the public that the certificate holder possesses the knowledge, skills, and experience to function effectively as a specialist in that area. The nature of the knowledge and skills to practice at a specialty level is subject to change due to technological and scientific advances. Recertification testing helps to provide continuing assurance that the certified specialist has indeed maintained knowledge in his or her specialty or focus area.

Therefore, those who wish to recertify in the same specialty area at the end of their 5-year certification period must meet the following criteria:

- Currently be a registered dietitian with the CDR
- Successfully complete an eligibility application
- Submit an application fee
- Provide documentation of the required minimum number of specialty practice hours
- Successfully complete a specialty examination

Appropriate Use of Credentials

In 1989, the CDR issued a statement on the protection of the credentials RD and DTR.[35] The CDR recognized that the credentials that it controls are most valuable to it and to the holders of those credentials because they are awarded only to individuals who have met the education and experiential requirements and have passed appropriate examinations. Practitioners may use these credentials only if they continue to meet CDR requirements, including payment of a registration maintenance fee and fulfillment of the continuing education hours required. The 2009 code of ethics for the profession of dietetics has specific details about the use of the various credentials of the Academy of Nutrition and Dietetics along with responsibilities and consequences.[36]

As noted in the CDR statement, "The most common usage is after the practitioner's name as a professional designation, e.g., Jane Doe, RD or John Smith, DTR."[37] Other specific details of the joint policy statement of the CDR and the academy's board of directors are included in the reference.[38]

LEGAL REGULATION OF DIETITIANS AND NUTRITIONISTS

Forty-six states now have laws that regulate dietitians or nutritionists through licensure, statutory certification, or registration. Thirty-one, or 67 percent, of these states have included the protection of a scope of practice as well as protection of the name registered dietitian; one half of these states protect the title of nutritionist as well; Nebraska protects the title of medical nutrition therapist, and Maine has licensure for dietetic technicians. State licensure and state certification are entirely separate and distinct from registration or certification by the CDR.

The 46 states that regulate dietitians or nutritionists do so through licensure, statutory certification, or registration. For state regulation purposes, these terms are defined as the following[39]:

- *Licensing.* Statutes include an explicitly defined scope of practice, and performance of the profession is illegal without first obtaining a license from the state.
- *Statutory certification.* Limits use of particular titles to persons meeting predetermined requirements, while persons not certified can still practice the occupation or profession.
- *Registration.* The least restrictive form of state regulation. As with certification, unregistered persons are permitted to practice the profession. Typically, exams are not given and enforcement of the registration requirement is minimal.

Dietetics practitioners are licensed by states to ensure that only qualified, trained professionals provide nutrition services or advice to individuals requiring or seeking nutrition care or dietetics information. In states with licensure, only state-licensed dietetics professionals can provide nutrition counseling and other services, included in the scope of practice, as a part of the licensure law. Nonlicensed practitioners may be subject to prosecution for practicing without a license. States with certification laws limit the use of particular titles (e.g., dietitian or nutritionist) to persons meeting predetermined requirements; however, persons not certified can still practice without using the title. Consumers in these states who are seeking nutrition therapy assistance need to be more cautious and aware of the qualifications of the provider they choose.

As dietitians or dietetic technicians travel from state to state to practice dietetics, it is important to contact a state regulatory agency to determine state licensure law provisions prior to practicing dietetics. State licensure agency contact information can usually be obtained by contacting the state dietetic association or the CDR, which maintains a current list of states with licensure or certification laws in place.

SUMMARY

Dietitians continue to desire recognition and differentiation among their peers that is visible and can be communicated to other professional practitioners. The credentialing program does this. The RD has become valued to the point that most individuals consider it synonymous with dietitian. The same is becoming true for the DTR. Many employers view both as mandatory credentials to practice in various employment settings. Credentials also have been used in international markets and jobs to describe individuals and job qualifications.[40] For dietitians, dietetic technicians, and dietetic specialists, this is a plus as the world moves toward a global practice and global economy.

Consumers will always demand credentials of some kind. As consumers recognize that the credentials of the ADA provide assurance that the practitioners are competent and can provide services they want, the demand will continue to rise. More significantly, these credentials will enhance the dietetics professionals' efforts to describe the diversity of their capabilities and to obtain a competitive advantage in the practice of dietetics in the United States and internationally.

DEFINITIONS

Certification. The process by which a nongovernmental agency or association grants recognition to an individual who has met certain predetermined qualifications specified by that agency or association (e.g., registration for dietitians and dietetic technicians administered by the CDR).

Credentialing. Formal recognition of professional or technical competence as by certification or licensure.

Licensure. Process by which a government agency grants permission to an individual to engage in a given occupation upon finding that the applicant has attained the minimal degree of competency necessary to ensure that the public health, safety, and welfare are reasonably well protected.

Practitioner. One who practices in a profession or occupation.

Registration. See Certification.

Scope of practice. Extent of or dimensions of activities performed in an area of practice.

REFERENCES

1. Needham, J. *Clerks and Craftsmen in China and the West. Lectures and Addresses on the History of the Science and Technology.* (Cambridge, MA: University Press, 1970), p. 95.
2. Cassell, J. *Carry the Flame: The History of the American Dietetic Association.* (Chicago: The American Dietetic Association, 1990), p. 9.
3. See Note 2, p. 3.
4. See Note 2, p. 22.
5. See Note 2, p. 26.
6. See Note 2, p. 71.
7. Perry, E. "Report of the Executive Board." *J Am Diet Assoc* 26 (1950): 949–957.
8. Bogle, M.L. "Registration: The *Sine Qua Non* of a Competent Dietitian." *J Am Diet Assoc* 74 (1974): 616–620.
9. ADA. *Constitution of the American Dietetic Association, as Amended.* (Chicago: The American Dietetic Association, 1971).
10. ADA. "Bylaws of American Dietetic Association," revised March 10, 2002. Accessed March 1, 2004, www.eatright.org/member/governance/85_12428.cfm
11. Wilson, A. "New Supervised Practice Pathway Offers Additional Options to Dietetics Graduates." *ADA Times* 9, no. 1 (2011, Autumn): 18–19.
12. O'Sullivan-Maillet, J., J. Skates, and E. Pritchett. "Scope of Dietetics Practice Framework." *J Am Diet Assoc* 105 (2005): 634–640.
13. ADA. "American Dietetic Association Revised 2008 Standards of Practice for Registered Dietitians in Nutrition Care; Standards of Professional Performance for Registered Dietitians; Standards of Practice for Dietetic Technicians, Registered; and Standards of Professional Performance for Dietetic Technicians, Registered." *J Am Diet Assoc* 108 (2008): 1535–1542.
14. ADA. *Final Report of the Phase 2 Future Practice and Education Task Force.* (Chicago: The American Dietetic Association, 2008), pp. 2–72.
15. ADA. "American Dietetic Association/Commission on Dietetic Registration Code of Ethics for the Profession of Dietetics and Process for Consideration of Ethics Issues." *J Am Diet Assoc* 109 (2009): 1461–1467.
16. ADA. *Council on Future Practice Visioning Report.* (Chicago: The American Dietetic Association, 2011).
17. Dreyfus, H.L., and S.E. Dreyfus. *Mind over Machine.* (New York: The Free Press, 1986).
18. See Note 12.
19. Dreyfus, S.E. "The Five-Stage Model of Adult Skill Acquisition." *Bull Sci Technol Soc* 14 (2004): 177–181.
20. Academy of Nutrition and Dietetics. "RD/DTR Credentialing (CDR)." Accessed October 10, 2012, http://www.eatright.org/HealthProfessionals/content.aspx?id=6442458781&terms=RD%2fDTR%20Credentialing#.UPsWAI5xBFA
21. See Note 19.

22. Benner, P. *From Novice to Expert*, Commemorative ed. (Upper Saddle River, NJ: Prentice Hall Health, 2001).

23. Bogle, M.L., L. Balogun, J. Cassell, A. Catakis, H.J. Holler, and C. Flynn. "Achieving Excellence in Dietetic Practice: Certification of Specialists and Advanced-Level Practitioners." *J Am Diet Assoc* 93 (1993): 149–150.

24. Bradley, R.T. "Fellow of the American Dietetic Association Credentialing Program: Development and Implementation of a Portfolio-Based Assessment." *J Am Diet Assoc* 96 (1996): 513–517.

25. Touger-Decker, R. "Advanced-Level Practice Degree Options: Practice Doctorates in Dietetics." *J Am Diet Assoc* 104 (2004): 1456–1458.

26. Skipper, A., and N.M. Lewis. "Using Initiative to Achieve Autonomy: A Model for Advanced Practice in Medical Nutrition Therapy." *J Am Diet Assoc* 106 (2006): 1219–1225.

27. See Note 15.

28. See Note 25.

29. Brody, R.A., L. Byham-Gray, M.R. Passannante, R. Touger-Decker, and J. O'Sullivan-Maillet. "Essential Practice Activities of Clinical Advanced Practice Registered Dietitians: A Delphi Study." *J Am Diet Assoc* 111 (2011): A17.

30. Brody, R.A., L. Byham-Gray, R. Touger-Decker, M.R. Passannante, and J. O'Sullivan Malliet. "Identifying Components of Advanced-Clinical Nutrition Practice: A Delphi Study." *J Am Diet Assoc* 112 (1012): 859–869.

31. Keirn, K.S., C.A. Johnson, and G.E. Gates. "Learning Needs and Continuing Professional Education Activities of Professional Development Portfolio Participants." *J Am Diet Assoc* 101, no. 6 (2001): 697–702.

32. Weddle, D.O., S.P. Himsburg, N. Collins, and R. Lewis. "The Professional Development Portfolio Process: Setting Goals for Credentialing." *J Am Diet Assoc* 102, no. 10 (2002): 1439–1444.

33. Dahl, L., and S. Nye. "Competency for Retired Credentialed Practitioners." *J Am Diet Assoc* 112 (2012): 934–936.

34. Keirn, K.S., G.E. Gates, and C.A. Johnson. "Dietetics Professionals Have a Positive Perception of Professional Development." *J Am Diet Assoc* 101, no. 7 (2001): 820–824.

35. Gates, G. "Ethics Opinion: Dietetic Professionals Are Ethically Obligated to Maintain Personal Competence in Practice." *J Am Diet Assoc* 103 (2003): 633–635.

36. See Note 15.

37. See Note 34.

38. See Note 34.

39. See Note 32.

40. See Note 32.

CHAPTER 5

The Nutrition and Dietetics Professional

"The dietetics practitioner provides professional services with objectivity and with respect for the unique needs and values of individuals."[1]

OUTLINE

- Introduction
- Scope of Practice and Standards of Practice
- Ethical Practice
- Culturally Competent Practice
- Lifelong Professional Development
  - Delivery of Learning
  - Informatics
- Legal Basis of Practice
- Evidence-Based Practice
- Public Policy Participation
- Summary
- Definitions
- References

INTRODUCTION

Professional practice can be defined in several ways—first and foremost, as practice based on specialized learning and training and adherence to a code of ethical actions adopted by the group. Dietitians who develop a professional portfolio are familiar with the process involved, such as a plan for continued competence in practice with supporting goals and measures to reach the goals. The portfolio emphasis is on continued learning and self-monitoring, both distinguishing features of a professional.

Dietetics practice is based on a fluid and flexible framework. The core of the profession is food and nutrition services for individuals, groups, and communities. The dietetics professional provides services through communication and collaboration with others by using management techniques, research, science, technology, and leadership skills.

SCOPE OF PRACTICE AND STANDARDS OF PRACTICE

In response to a need to provide guidance for members practicing in diverse roles in dietetics, the ADA appointed a task force in 2004 to develop a scope of dietetics practice framework (SDPF). Completed in 2005, directions for usage of the framework by members followed in 2006.[2,3] It was updated in 2011 by a committee of the house of delegates (HOD).[4] The framework provides a flexible decision-making structure by which practitioners can determine if specific activities fall within the scope of dietetics practice. The following three broad areas are defined in the framework: foundation knowledge, evaluation, and resources.

Among the 46 states that have enacted state licensure, many include a scope of practice definition patterned after the national document. Such guidelines help define practice for legislators and give direction to dietitians practicing in a particular state.

The ADA first published guidelines for professional practice in 1998.[5] In 2003, they were replaced by the standards of professional performance (SOPP) to more accurately describe their content and function.[6] Standards of performance (SOP) have also been developed in many areas of dietetics practice. These are complementary documents. The SOP describes a skills competence level of behavior in the professional role. Together, they serve to describe the practice and performance of dietitians and dietetic technicians.

The first standards for a specific area of practice were developed in 2005 in nutrition care[7] and updated in 2008.[8] They were general standards in that they outline activities that apply in all areas of dietetics practice. They have become the blueprint for the development of standards in many other areas of practice.

The general standards provide for the following activities:

- Describing minimum levels of practice and performance
- Providing common indicators for self-evaluation
- Promoting consistency in practice and performance
- Describing the role of dietetics and the unique services that RDs and DTRs provide within the healthcare team
- Illustrating that food and nutrition services are provided in a framework that encourages continuous quality improvement
- Providing a basis for researchers to investigate relationships between dietetics practice and outcomes
- Providing a framework for educators to set objectives for educational programs that reflect applicable federal laws and regulations

Standards are important for the following reasons:

- They promote safe, effective, and efficient food and nutrition services.
- They are based on evidence-based practice.
- They provide for improved health care and food and nutrition service-related outcomes.
- They ensure continuous quality improvement.
- They promote dietetics research, innovation, and practice development.
- They help the individual RD and DTR develop professionally.

Specific standards that have been developed in several areas of practice include the following: nutrition care,[9] nutrition support,[10] behavioral health care,[11] management,[12] education of dietetic practitioners,[13] sports dietetics,[14] diabetes care,[15] oncology,[16] integrative and functional medicine,[17] disordered eating and eating disorders,[18] extended care,[19] pediatric nutrition,[20] and nephrology care.[21]

In addition to becoming proficient in an area of practice and continually monitoring performance, there are related areas of knowledge and practice that support and enhance competence but are not generally evident in a job description. Specifically, the areas discussed in this chapter include ethical practice, lifelong professional development, the legal basis practice, political awareness, evidence-based practice, and issues related to diversity.

ETHICAL PRACTICE

The professional code of ethics[22] is the guiding document for ethical practice in dietetics. The framework in which such policies are developed is the hallmark of an effective structure that includes the following[23]:

- Guiding values and commitments are sensible and clearly communicated.
- Organizational leaders are personally committed, credible, and willing to take action on the values they espouse.
- Values are integrated into the normal channels of management decision making and are reflected in the organization's critical activities.
- The organization's systems and structures support and enforce its values.
- Managers throughout the organization have the decision-making skill, knowledge, and competence needed to make ethically sound decisions on a day-to-day basis.

In practice, situations arise at times in which it is not always clear what the ethical course of action should be. Ethical conflicts of interest and poorly conducted business practices are examples of how ethical conduct impacts dietetic practice.[24–27] Other ethical considerations include issues of confidentiality, promotion and endorsement of products, and recognition of professional judgment.

In clinical practice, activities relating to dispensing dietary supplementation advice and conducting online counseling and consultation make it important to be familiar with regulations as well as the code of ethics in order to avoid liability risk. Other instances in which ethical conduct must be considered are disclosure of confidential information, accepting gifts, discussing patients, charting, or giving information about prices or salaries. In such cases, open discussion with a supervisor or trusted peers before action is the best course to follow. A personal code of conduct that espouses integrity, fairness, and a sense of always wanting to do the right thing helps make difficult decisions about ethical questions easier. The manager or leader assists in developing organization practices and policies that promote ethical practice. Such policies set the ethical standards for purchasing, financial management, patient care issues, information provided to patients, and clients. The manager or leader sets an example for ethical behavior built on openness and trust. An ethical deliberation process is shown in **Table 5-1**.

Table 5-1. Suggested Ethical Deliberative Process

1. Clarify the moral question—the first statement of the moral problem.
2. Re-create the context.
   a. Gather data.
   b. Consider relevant facts.
   c. Consider relevant values.
3. Name stakeholders and their relationships.
4. Identify ways of ethical thinking used by the stakeholders.
   a. *Rules thinking*—doing what is right by following the rules
   b. *Roles thinking*—being true to self and your sense of virtue
   c. *Goals thinking*—producing good outcomes regardless of rules
5. Determine practical limits to the situation: policies, laws, standards, and codes.
6. Balance a client's beliefs and preferences with his or her best interests.
7. Respect advance directives.
8. Assume a client has decisional capacity.
9. If not, select a substitute decision maker if necessary.
10. Restate the ethical problem.
11. Search for possible options.
12. Test various options. Check through each option for:
    a. *Rules*—is it right?
    b. *Roles*—can I feel good about this?
    c. *Goals*—what good will it do?
13. Justify the option selected for recommendation.
    a. Keep the client's best interest at the center of options.
    b. Provide a description of what will likely happen and provide a clear action.
    c. Plan for each option recommended—suggestions of practical pathways.

Source: Reprinted from Journal of the American Dietetic Association, 102, Number 5 (May 2002): Julie O'Sullivan Maillet et al, "Position of the American Dietetic Association: Ethical and Legal Issues in Nutrition, Hydration, and Feeding," 716–726, Copyright 2002, with permission from Elsevier.

The increased use of electronic communications in all areas of practice demands ethical decision making.[28] Much of the communication is through use of social networks, such as Facebook, LinkedIn, Twitter, blogs, etc., as well as cell phones and tablet computers. There are no guidelines for the use of these forms of media that deal with ethical behavior and communications with the public, and it is often difficult to tell what is reliable and valid information. The Nutrition Entrepreneurs Dietetic Practice Group has established a nutrition blog network to make it easier to find science-based information and elevate the voice of registered dietitians online.[29] *E-professionalism* is a term used to describe professional attitudes and behaviors in the use of digital media and applies to still-evolving standards of practice, legality, etiquette, and perception.[30]

Ethics in research and in the use of copyrighted research from journals are further areas in which dietitians are obligated to follow practices of honesty, fairness, and integrity and to avoid conflict of interest and any action affecting professional judgment in conducting industry-funded research.[31,32]

The ADA *Code of Ethics for the Profession of Dietetics* has been revised and adapted by the ADA and the CDR as a voluntary enforceable code of behavior. The code challenges all members to uphold ethical principles. The process of enforcement includes a system to deal with any complaint about members and credentialed practitioners. The ethics committee enforces the code and educates members about the ethical principles to be followed.

CULTURALLY COMPETENT PRACTICE

A former president of the ADA described culturally competent practice as a way to overcome health disparities and improve care across all population groups.[33] Interaction with clients of diverse cultures in a sensitive and effective manner is a key strategy in the promotion of food and nutrition behavior and beliefs.

The way many institutions and groups implement plans for ensuring cultural competence is through diversity initiatives. Diversity can refer to age, physical ability, religion, socioeconomic status, sex, and ethnicity. Associations often focus on attracting a membership that reflects these demographics. The Academy, however, has developed a number of initiatives toward promoting diversity including an official statement:

> The Academy's values and respects the diverse viewpoints and individual difference of all people. The Academy's mission and vision are most effectively realized through the promotion of a diverse membership that reflects cultural, ethnic, gender, racial, religious, sexual orientation, socioeconomic, geographical, political, educational, experiential and philosophical characteristics of the public it serves. The Academy actively identifies and offers opportunities to individuals with varied skills, talents, abilities, ideas, disabilities, backgrounds and practice expertise.[34]

A template for creating a diversity plan was published in the journal in 2011,[35] as was a set of principles from the code of ethics relating to ensuring equality in practice.[36]

LIFELONG PROFESSIONAL DEVELOPMENT

The Center for Professional Development in the academy office offers and coordinates many activities designed to support all food and nutrition professionals in continual building of their knowledge and skills through multidisciplinary activities, enhanced technology, and programming. Examples are the annual Food and Nutrition Conference and Exposition (FNCE); training programs for specialty certification; and conferences and events, including sessions at the FNCE conducted by the dietetic practice groups. Distance learning opportunities are also offered through teleseminars and webinars. In addition, group and individual self-study is available.

A plan was implemented to improve compensation levels through professional development activities by the ADA.[37] The Performance, Proficiency, and Value Plan had the goals of using various approaches to close the gaps between performance, proficiency, and value and that members would adopt various approaches to enhance personal value. Many positive benefits have come from the undertaking, both professionally and through increased compensation levels.

Delivery of Learning

Food and nutrition professionals use a variety of methods to continually build their knowledge and skills. The range of learning opportunities is greater than ever considering the many advancements in technology that allow individual study as well as group learning and interaction. For instance, teleconferencing today replaces many former face-to-face meetings, thus saving travel and related costs. Networking through social network sites is fast becoming a way for dietetic professionals to connect with and learn from others with similar interests and concerns.[38,39]

Technologies often used in distance education are *synchronous* (participants meet together) or *asynchronous* (participants access information at their own convenience). Examples of synchronous methods are individual and conference calls, videoconferences and web conferences. Asynchronous methods include audiocassettes, e-mail, message boards, print materials, voice mail, fax, CDs, and videocassettes. Distance education courses are offered in several ways: by correspondence through regular mail; through the Internet, through telecourses in which content is delivered by radio or television; CD-ROM instruction in which the student interacts with computer content stored in the file; pocket/mobile learning through mobile devices or wireless service; and integrated learning through in-group instruction with a distance learning curriculum.

Online video and streaming video have proven to be effective ways of communicating nutrition messages.[40] Switt[41] offers suggestions for creating and managing a website by offering unique, original content; registering with search engines; and developing a newsletter.

Self-direction in learning is the ability to engage in educational activities without external reinforcement. Individuals who do so embody some or all of the following characteristics:

- Willingness to change
- Ability to identify weaknesses or shortcomings
- Ability to capitalize on strengths and passions
- Ability to experience learning from constructive criticism
- Willingness to participate in all forms of learning
- Willingness to try new techniques for learning
- Willingness to invest one's time and money in learning
- Willingness to find a mentor or become one
- Volunteering in organizations and groups
- Sharing learning by applying concepts and discussing with others
- Providing feedback to instructors, mentors, and supervisors
- Assuming individual responsibility for learning
- Allowing the possibility of new careers and experiences

Besides maintaining and improving professional competence, there are other reasons why practitioners participate in continuing education activities and why there may be deterrents in doing so. Several reasons and deterrents are shown in **Table 5-2**.

To determine the types of learning experiences that most benefit an individual, several questions may be posed for self-examination of needs (**Table 5-3**).

Informatics

Informatics is the fast-growing area of electronic support for using and managing information. Health informatics is described by the Department of Health and Human Services as the intersection of information science, computer media, and health care. Health information tools include electronic media, clinical guidelines, formal medical terminologies, and information and communication systems. The medical and nursing professions have taken the lead in the use of the technology, most directly in the development of electronic health records.[42]

Nutrition informatics is defined as "the effective retrieval, organization, storage, and optimum use of information, data, and knowledge of food

---

Table 5-2. Factors Influencing Continuing Professional Education

Reasons for participation in continuing professional education:
- Professional development and improvement
- Professional service
- Collegial learning and interaction
- Professional commitment and reflection
- Personal benefits and job security

Deterrents to participation in continuing professional education:
- Disengagement and apathy for learning or career
- Costs
- Family
- Failure to see the worth or benefit
- Lack of quality in offerings
- Demands of work constraints

Source: Reprinted from Journal of the American Dietetic Association, 103, Number 3 (March 2003), Petrillo, T. "Lifelong Learning Goals: Individual Steps That Propel the Profession of Dietetics," 298–300, Copyright 2003, with permission from Elsevier.

Table 5-3. Questions to Determine Self-Needs

What kind of learning is needed to improve performance in your current job?
How can you change or improve your current job?
What is your capacity for learning and growth in a new job?
What transferable skills do you possess for a new career path?
What new skills are required for you to be qualified to contribute in a new job?
What are your personal interests?
What career paths did you once consider?
What leisure time interests do you enjoy?
What type of a learning experience is most favorable to you and why?
What related learning opportunities lie just beyond your field of practice?
What skill sets are important to your employer?

Sources: Data from Davis, J.R. *Toolbox for Reflection and Developing an Action Learning Plan: Managing Your Own.* (San Francisco: Berrett-Koehler Publisher 2000), p. 10.
Petrillo, T. "Lifelong Learning Goals: Individual Steps That Propel the Profession of Dietetics." *J Am Diet Assoc* 103, no. 3 (2003): 298–300.

and nutrition-related problem solving and decision making. Informatics is supported by the use of information standards, information processes, and information technology."[43] The term is also defined simply as the intersection of information, nutrition, and technology. The use of automation is transforming dietetic practice in hospital dietary departments as well as in business, research, and private practice. The time involved in nutrition assessments of patients can be considerably decreased, communications between clinical and food service areas can be accomplished much faster, and dietitians have the opportunity to help shape the trend toward total automation in hospitals and food service institutions. The demand for informatics is expected to continue to grow, making this an area in which dietitians need to become proficient, perhaps through continued education.[44]

Graham has pointed out that dietitians should use websites for information that is scientifically sound and that many sites provide comprehensive coverage from multiple sources.[45] Among these are the ADA Evidence Analysis Library (www.andevidence.library.com).

The extent to which members use technology and for what purposes was surveyed in 2008 and again in 2011.[46] Both active members and students responded to the survey. Over half the respondents indicated they strongly agreed with a statement that they used data and technology to solve problems. Slightly fewer (45%) strongly agreed they use data and technology to make decisions. Among 10 categories of uses of technology, there was an increase in the usage of every type, with a threefold increase in use of webinars. This very likely reflects the availability of more programs offered by the academy, as well as from other sources, for continuing education.

All practitioners need to be familiar with the provisions of the Health Insurance Portability and Accountability Act of 1996 (HIPAA) and the further Privacy Rule of 2003.[47] Developed by the Department of Health and Human Services, these acts provide patients with access to their medical records and more control over how their personal health information is used and disclosed. HIPAA includes provisions for electronic transactions and safeguards to protect the security and confidentiality of health information. All health providers, including dietitians, must be aware of the need to protect the privacy of information about patients in the clinical setting and become familiar with the policies and procedures established by the institution for the enforcement of the regulations.[48]

A national undertaking that will connect health records to electronics for every American by 2014 is under way.[49] The dietetics profession is a part of this national effort, making it imperative that a concerted effort is made to prepare practitioners for the use of nutrition information aligned with the broad fields of medicine and health. This also presents the opportunity to integrate food and nutrition with related activities into the system.

LEGAL BASIS OF PRACTICE

The practice of dietetics is directly affected by many laws and regulations that must be followed in order to avoid legal consequences. Fortunately, as Derelian[50] points out, almost all disputes that include a dietitian would be of a civil nature, such as contract breaches or negligence. Busey[51] indicates that dietitians may increasingly become parties to lawsuits considering the number of RDs who go into private practice and the fact that RDs play important roles in the healthcare process. He gives suggestions regarding the types of lawsuits in which a dietitian may become involved and discusses steps in the process when lawsuits occur. He further points out that if the terminology used in documentation of patient care is subject to more than one interpretation, this could become a legally disputed issue. An example is the use of the word *inadequate* in describing patient progress, as it could denote negligence.[52]

The greater use of electronic technology such as in telehealth or telemedicine in which a dietitian may be a participant is another area in which legal questions may arise.[53] Examples of issues that may apply are licensure, facility certification and accreditation, reimbursement and Medicare Part B issues, and professional liability issuance. All dietitians are strongly encouraged to carry personal liability insurance for protection against malpractice or issues such as those described previously.

EVIDENCE-BASED PRACTICE

Evidence-based practice (EBP) is viewed as necessary for the best outcomes in all areas of dietetic practice. Evidence-based medicine is a model of clinical decision making that uses a systematic process to integrate the best research-based evidence with clinical expertise and patient values to answer a question about a patient's plan of care in order to optimize outcomes.[54] In dietetics, EBP can be described a process by which the best available data are consulted to make decisions, followed by evaluation of the outcome of these decisions.[55] Dietitians need to incorporate EBP into all activities and decisions. Payment for services may be dependent on outcomes, because change in practice is constant, and this approach ensures that decisions are sound. By applying this process, dietitians are able to successfully compete in the healthcare environment where positive outcomes, proven efficiency, cost effectiveness, and sharing of outcomes are important. The healthcare manager, who may be the dietitian in charge, is often the catalyst for assuring that evidence-based information is integrated into healthcare management decisions.[56]

The academy provides a valuable resource to members through the Evidence Analysis Library (EAL). Through the EAL process outlined, professionals can stay up to date on the research in all areas of dietetics. A variety of resources are offered, including evidence summaries of the major research on a given topic, bibliographies, and conclusion statements with an evaluation of the strength of he evidence.[57]

A guide for appraising resources for evidence-based information is shown in **Table 5-4**. Evidence must be balanced with the client's values

Table 5-4. Guide for Appraising Resources for Evidence-Based Information

Methods and quality of information
- How was the resource compiled?
- Were explicit criteria for seeking and appraising evidence described, and were they adhered to?
- How is the resource maintained?

Rating scale for methods and quality of information

0 No evidence cited

1 Evidence is cited, but there are no explicit criteria for the selection or the evaluation of the content; the election of content suggests lack of consistent evidence standards.

2 Evidence is cited, and there are explicit criteria for the selection or evaluation of the content, or both; the selection of content suggests lack of adherence to these evidence standards.

3 Evidence is cited, but there are no explicit criteria for the selection or evaluation of the content; the selection of content suggest adherence to some evidence standards.

4 Evidence is cited, and there are explicit criteria for the selection or evaluation of the content, or both; the selection of content suggests some adherence to evidence standards.

5 Evidence is cited, and there are explicit criteria for the selection and evaluation of the content; the selection of content suggests adherence to evidence standards most of the time.

Clinical usefulness
- Did the resource provide clinically useful answers?
- How did you use this resource?
- Was it easy to use?
- Were the answers easily accessible and readable within a few minutes?
- Will you use this resource?
- If so, when and how?

Rating scale for clinical usefulness

0 Not useful clinically.

1 Clinically useful answers are rarely available and are not easily accessible or readable within a few minutes.

2 Clinically useful answers are available some of the time but are not easily accessible or readable within a few minutes.

3 Clinically useful answers are available some of the time and are easily accessible and readable within a few minutes.

4 Clinically useful answers are available most of the time but are not easily accessible or readable within a few minutes.

5 Clinically useful answers are available most of the time and are easily accessible and readable within a few minutes.

(continues)

Table 5-4. Guide for Appraising Resources for Evidence-Based Information *(continued)*

Details on specific resources

Evidence-based medical texts

The following points could be used as a minimal checklist:

- Does the resource provide an explicit statement about the type of evidence on which any statements or recommendations are based? Did the authors adhere to these criteria? For example, claims about effectiveness of an intervention might be accompanied by a statement about either the level of evidence (which would need to be defined somewhere in the text) or a statement about the exact type of evidence (e.g., "There have been three randomized controlled trials.").

- Was there an explicit and adequate search for this evidence? For example, a search for evidence about an intervention might have started with a look for adequate systematic reviews. If this was done, it might be followed by a search of the Cochrane Central Register of Controlled Trials.

- Is there quantification of the results? For example, statements about diagnostic accuracy should contain measures of accuracy such as sensitivity and specificity.

The minimum criteria for an evidence-based resource would be adherence to the first bullet point. Better resources should also address the other two points.

Meta-resources (e.g., listings or search engines for other resources)

These resources should provide an explicit statement about the selection criteria for inclusion in the listing. Better resources should also include a descriptive review such as that described in the three points for evidence-based medical texts.

Source: Straus, S., and R.B. Haynes. "Managing Evidence-Based Knowledge: The Need for Reliable, Relevant, and Readable Resources." CMAJ 180, no. 9(2009): 942–945. Copyright © 2009. This work is protected by copyright and the making of this copy was with the permission of Access Copyright. Any alteration of its content or further copying in any form whatsoever is strictly prohibited unless otherwise permitted by law.

and preferences for optimal shared decision-making, and information resources must be reliable, relevant, and readable.[58]

PUBLIC POLICY PARTICIPATION

Each year, the Legislative and Public Policy Committee of the academy, under the direction of the board of directors, establishes policy priorities based on member and association interests and legislation under consideration at the national level. The priority areas in which the academy works from year to year include food and food safety, healthcare reform, health literacy and nutrition advancement, medical nutrition therapy, aging, child nutrition, Medicaid and Medicare, nutrition monitoring and research, obesity, and healthy weight management.

The priority areas in which the academy was working in 2012 were the following:

1. *Aging.* Nutrition practices affect functionality and the quality of life in older adults. Medical nutrition therapy helps manage chronic diseases and slows their progression. The goal is to assist older adults to remain independent longer and enjoy the benefits of good health.

2. *Child nutrition.* Food and nutrition programs provide access to a safe, nutritious, and adequate food supply while nutrition screening and assessment are important for child and adolescent health and well-being.

3. *Food and food safety.* Collaboration with the government agencies (primarily the Food and Drug Administration and the U.S. Department of Agriculture) that regulate foods and food safety leads to better public education as well as setting the agenda for policy decisions.

4. *Health literacy and nutrition advancement.* The promotion of a healthful eating style that emphasizes balance in the total diet, combined with moderation in intake and physical activity, is the goal of dietetics professionals.

5. *Healthy, Hunger-Free Kids Act of 2010.* Enacted by the Senate, this child nutrition reauthorization act provides for changes in child nutrition through healthier meal options.

6. *Medical Nutrition Therapy and Medicare/Medicaid.* The academy seeks to enlarge the scope of medical nutrition therapy for management of specific disease states. The cost-effectiveness of medical nutrition therapy has been demonstrated, and the authorization of its further use would result in reductions in incidence and severity of diseases.

7. *Nutrition monitoring and research.* Information about what Americans eat allows for nutrition education directed toward helping consumers make the connection between diet and health.

8. *Obesity/overweight/healthy weight management.* The prevalence of overweight and obesity among all segments of the population is an ongoing concern through their impact on health as well as on the cost of treating their complications.

Both federal and state policies affect dietetic practice in many ways. As noted earlier, credentialing and state licensure are authorized by governmental action. Dietitians who work in hospitals, nursing homes, assisted living facilities, nursing facilities, renal dialysis facilities, and home health programs must follow state regulations governing these programs. The Centers for Medicare & Medicaid Services specify the kind of dietary services to be provided and the eligibility of those working in the programs.[59] Because almost all practice areas are governed by laws and regulations in various ways, dietitians must not only be aware of the requirements but also have opportunities for providing input into how they affect practice. This can happen several ways through state efforts and a national conference each year. The academy provides materials to use in advocacy efforts and maintains a political action committee (PAC).

SUMMARY

The professional dietitian is one who is competent in practice and continually participates in ongoing education. Knowledge and skills go hand in hand with personal qualities and practice, including ethical practice, awareness of government influence, understanding of the legal basis of practice, and incorporating the concept of evidence-based activities into professional practice. As the voice of authority in food and nutrition, the dietitian is a professional in every sense of the term.

DEFINITIONS

Evidence based. Action based on research data and evaluation of outcomes.

Profession. An occupation that involves specialized knowledge and training in which members subscribe to group beliefs and practices.

Public policy. A course of action by a government entity.

Regulation. A written directive that implements a law.

REFERENCES

1. American Dietetic Association/Commission on Dietetic Registration. "Code of Ethics for the Profession of Dietetics and Process for Consideration of Ethics Issues." *J Am Diet Assoc* 109, no. 9 (2009): 1461–1467.
2. Maillet, J., J. Skates, and E. Pritchett. "American Dietetic Association: Scope of Dietetics Practice Framework." *J Am Diet Assoc* 105, no.4 (2005): 634–640.

3 Viscooan, B., and J. 3wltt. "Undertaking and Using the Scope of Dietetics Practice Framework: A Step-Wise approach." *J Am Diet Assoc* 106, no. 3 (2006): 459–463.

4. Academy of Nutrition and Dietetics. "Scope of Dietetics Practice Framework Defined." Accessed March 2, 2012, www.eatright.org

5. ADA. "The American Dietetic Association Standards of Professional Practice for Dietetics Professionals." *J Am Diet Assoc* 98, no. 1 (1998): 83–87.

6. Kieselhorst, K.J., J. Skates, and E. Pritchett. "American Dietetic Association Standards of Practice in Nutrition Care and Updated Standards of Professional Performance." *J Am Diet Assoc* 105, no. 4 (2005): 641–645.

7. See Note 6.

8. American Dietetic Association Quality Management Committee. "American Dietetic Association Revised 2008 Standards of Practice for Registered Dietitians in Nutrition Care; Standards of Professional Performance for Registered Dietitians; Standards of Practice for Dietetic Technicians, Registered, in Nutrition Care; and Standards of Professional Performance for Dietetic Technicians, Registered." *J Am Diet Assoc* 108, no. 9 (2008): 1538–1542.

9. See Note 8.

10. The Joint Standards Task Force of A.S.P.E.N. and the American Dietetic Association Dietitians in Nutrition Support Dietetic Practice Group. "The American Society for Parenteral and Enteral Nutrition and the American Dietetic Association: Standards of Practice and Standards of Professional Performance for Registered Dietitians (Generalist, Specialty, and Advanced) in Nutrition Support." *J Am Diet Assoc* 107, no. 10 (2007): 1815–1822.

11. Emerson, M., P. Kerr, M.D.C. Soler, T.A. Girard, R. Hoffinger, E. Pritchett, and M. Otto. "American Dietetic Association Standards of Practice and Standards of Professional Performance for Registered Dietitians (Generalist, Specialty, and Advanced) in Behavioral Health Care." *J Am Diet Assoc* 106, no. 6 (2006): 608–613.

12. Puckett, R.P., M. Barkley, G. Dixon, K. Egan, C. Koch, T. Malone, J. Scott-Smith, B. Sheridan, and M. Theis. "American Dietetic Association: Standards of Professional Performance for Registered Dietitians (Generalist and Advanced) in Management of Food and Nutrition Systems." *J Am Diet Assoc* 109, no. 3 (2009): 540–552.

13. Anderson, J.A., K. Kennedy-Hagen, M.R. Stieber, D.S. Hollingsworth, K. Kattelmann, C.L. Stein Arnold, and B.M. Egan. "Dietetic Educators of Practitioners and American Dietetic Association Standards of Professional Performance for Registered Dietitians (Generalist, Specialty/Advanced) in Education of Dietetics Practitioners." *J Am Diet Assoc* 109, no. 4 (2009): 747–754.

14. Bteinmuller, P.L., N.L. Meyer, L.K. Fruskall, M.N. Manore, N.R. Rodriguez, M. Macedonio, R., L. Bird, and J.R. Berning. "American Dietetic Association Standards of Practice and Standards of Professional Performance for Registered Dietitians (Generalist, Specialty, Advanced) in Sports Dietetics." *J Am Diet Assoc* 109, no. 3 (2009): 544–551.

15. Boucher, J.L., A. Evert, A. Daly, K. Kulkarni, J. Rizzotto, K. Burton, and B.G. Bradshaw. "American Dietetic Association Revised Standards of Practice and Standards of Professional Performance for Registered Dietitians (Generalist, Specialty, and Advanced) in Diabetes Care." *J Am Diet Assoc* 111, no. 1 (2011): 156–166.

16. Robien, K., L. Bechard, L. Elliott, N. Fox, R. Levin, and S. Washburn. "American Dietetic Association: Revised Standards of Practice and Standards of Professional Performance for Registered Dietitians (Generalist, Specialty, and Advanced) in Oncology Nutrition Care." *J Am Diet Assoc* 110, no. 2 (2010): 310–317.

17. Ford, D., R. Sudha, R.K. Batheja, R. DeBusk, D. Grotto, D. Noland, E. Redmond, and K.M. Swift. "American Dietetic Association: Standards of Practice and Standards of Professional Performance for Registered Dietitians (Competent, Proficient, and Expert) in Integrative and Functional Medicine." *J Am Diet Assoc* 111, no. 8 (2011): 902–911.

18. Tholking, M.M., A.C. Mellowspring, S.G. Eberle, R.P. Lamb, E.S. Myers, C. Scribner, R.F. Sloan, and K.B. Wetherall. "American Dietetic Association: Standards of Practice and Standards of Professional Performance for Registered Dietitians (Competent, Proficient, and Expert) in Disordered Eating and Eating Disorders (DE and ED)." *J Am Diet Assoc* 111, no. 9 (2011): 1242–1249.

19. Roberts, L., S.C. Cryst, G.E. Robinson, C.H. Elliott, L.C. Moore, M. Rybicki, and M.P. Carlson. "American Dietetic Association: Standards of Practice and Standards of Professional Performance for Registered Dietitians (Competent, Proficient, and Expert) in Extended Care Settings." *J Am Diet Assoc* 111, no. 4 (2011): 617–624.

20. Charney, P., B. Ogata, N. Nevin-Folino, K. Holt, H. Brewer, M.K. Sharett, and L.A. Carney. "American Dietetic Association: Standards of Practice and Standards of Professional Performance (Generalist, Specialty, and Advanced) for Registered Dietiians in Pediatric Nutrition." *J Am Diet Assoc* 109 (2009): 1468–1478.

21. Brommage, D., M. Karalis, C. Martin, M. McCarthy, D. Benner, C.M. Goeddeke-Merickel, K.Wiesen, et al. "American Dietetic Association and the National Kidney Foundation Standards of Practice and Standards of Professional Performance for Registered Dietitians (Generalist, Specialty, and Advanced) in Nephrology Care." *J Am Diet Assoc* 109 (2009): 1617–1625.

22. American Dietetic Association/Commission on Dietetic Registration. "Code of Ethics for the Profession of Dietetics." *J Am Diet Assoc* 109, no. 8 (2009): 1461–1467.

23. Paine, L.S. "Managing for Organizational Integrity." *Harvard Business Review* 72 (1994): 106–117.

24. Waynack, M.H. "Ethical Conflicts of Interest." *J Am Diet Assoc* 103, no. 5 (2003): 555–557.

25. Fornari, A. "Professional Boundary Issues in Practice." *J Am Diet Assoc* 103, no. 3 (2003): 380.

26. Grandgenett, R., and D. Derelian. "Ethics in Business Practice." *J Am Diet Assoc* 110, no. 7 (2010): 1103–1104.

27. Fuhrman, M.P. "Issues Facing Dietetics Professionals: Challenges and Opportunities." *J Am Diet Assoc* 102, no. 11 (2002): 1618–1620.

28. Castle, D., and R. DeBusk. "The Electronic Health Record: Genetic Information and Patient Privacy." *J Am Diet Assoc* 108, no. 8 (2008): 1372–1374.

29. Ventures, Newsletter of Nutrition Entrepreneurs DPG. "Nutrition Blog Network." *Acad Nut and Diet* XXXVII, no. 1 (2010, Summer): p. 2.

30. Aase, S. "Toward E-Professionalism; Thinking Through the Implications of Navigating the Digital World." *J Am Diet Assoc* 110, no. 10 (2010): 1442–1449.

31. See Note 29.

32. Nicklas, T.A., W. Karmally, and C.E. O'Neil. "Nutrition Professionals Are Obligated to Follow Ethical Guidelines When Conducting Industry-Funded Research." *J Am Diet Assoc* 111, no. 12 (2011): 1931–1932.

33. Rodriguez, J.C. "Culturally Competent Dietetics: Increasing Awareness, Improving Care." *J Am Diet Assoc* 119, no. 5 (2010): S7.

34. Stein, K. "The Balancing Act of Diversity Initiatives." *J Am Diet Assoc* 111, no. 8 (2011): 1110–1117.

35. See Note 34.

36. Ethics Committee, American Dietetic Association. "Ethics: Opinion; Eliminating Dietetics-Related Inequalities." *J Am Diet Assoc* 111, no. 2 (2011): 307–309.

37. American Dietetic Association. 2005–2006 Ethics Committee. "Performance, Proficiency, and Value of the Dietetics Professional: An Update." *J Am Diet Assoc* 103, no. 10 (2003): 1376–1379.

38. Graham, L.K. "What Is Social Networking and How Do I Get Clued in to LinkedIn?" *J Am Diet Assoc* 109, no. 1 (2009): 184.

39. Brown, D. "Networking Moves. Online." *J Am Diet Assoc* 109, no. 2 (2009): 210–211.

40. Lane, M. "Streaming Soon to a Computer Near You: How Online Video Will Change Media and Maybe Your Practice Forever." *ADA Times* 5, no. 1 (2007): 12–15.

41. Switt, J.T. "Drawing Attention to Your Web Site." *J Am Diet Assoc* 108, no. 1 (2008): 20.

42. Hoggle, L.B., M.A. Michael, S.M. Houston, and E.J. Ayres. "Nutrition Informatics." *J Am Diet Assoc* 108, no. 1 (2008): 134–139.

43. Yadrick, M.M. "Informatics: A Word We Need to Know." [President's page]. *J Am Diet Assoc* 108, no. 1 (2008): 1976.

44. Aase, Y. "Improved Understanding the Promises and Challenges Nutrition Informatics Poses for Dietetics Careers." *J Am Diet Assoc* 110, no. 12 (2010): 1794–1798.

45. Graham, L. "Searching for Health Information: Web Sites and Tips for Finding Science-Based Sources." *J Am Diet Assoc* 110, no. 4 (2010): 513–514.

46. Ayres, E.J. "Nutrition Informatics Member Survey." *Acad Nutr Diet J* 2012 (112), no. 3 (2010): 360–367.
47. U.S. Department of Health and Human Services. "Understanding Health Information Privacy." Accessed April 15, 2012, www.hhs.gov/ocr/privacy/hipaa /understanding/
48. Hoggle, L.B., M.A. Michael, S.M. Houston, and E.J. Ayres. "Electronic Health Record: Where Does Nutrition Fit In?" *J Am Diet Assoc* 106, no. 10 (2006): 1688–1695.
49. See Note 48.
50. Derelian, D. "Dietetics; Legalities, Ethics, and Eccentricities." *J Am Diet Assoc* 100, no. 5 (2000): 519–523.
51. Busey, J.C. "Help! I've Just Been Served with a Lawsuit." *J Am Diet Assoc* 109, no. 4 (2009): 600–605.
52. Busey, J.C. "Use of the Word Inadequate—A Legal Perspective." *J Am Diet Assoc* 108, no. 6 (2008): 935–936.
53. Busey, J.C. "Telehealth—Opportunities and Pitfalls." *J Am Diet Assoc* 108, no. 8 (2008): 1296–1301.
54. Shanklin, C. "Evidence-Based Practice: Practice Based on Evidence, Right?" *ADA Times* 1, no. 3 (2003): 1, 3.
55. Blumberg-Kason, S. "Evidence-Based Nutrition Practice Guidelines: A Valuable Resource in the Evidence Analysis Library." *J Am Diet Assoc* 106, no. 12 (2006): 1935–1936.
56. Smith, K.P.D., and J. Woods. "The Healthcare Manager as Catalyst for Evidence-Based Practice: Changing the Healthcare Environment and Changing Experience." *Healthcare Papers* 300, no. 3 (2003): 54–57.
57. Academy of Nutrition and Dietetics. "Evidence Based Practice." Accessed April 1, 2012, www.eatright.org
58. Straus, S., and R.B. Haynes. "Managing Evidence-Based Knowledge: The Need for Reliable, Relevant and Readable Resources." *CMAJ* 180, no. 9 (2009): 942–945.
59. Whitley, D.L. "Setting the Standard: Including the RD and DTR in State Facility Policies." *J Am Diet Assoc* 110, no. 5 (2010): 687–688.

The Dietitian in Clinical Practice

"We need both cognitive ability and emotional intelligence to help people understand and use the Dietary Guidelines."[1]

OUTLINE

- · Summary
- · Definitions
- · References

INTRODUCTION

The discipline of clinical dietetics originated in 1899 when *dietitian* was defined by the American Home Economics Association as "individuals with a knowledge of food who provide diet therapy for the medical profession."[2] Until 1917, dietitians were affiliated with this association, but after 1917 they belonged to the newly formed American Dietetic Association.[3]

The earliest dietitians worked primarily in hospitals or were associated with food assistance programs. During the 1930s and 1940s, dietitians became involved in either food production and food service or in the planning and provision of diets for special medical needs. The title, *therapeutic dietitian*, was used to describe the person who provided food for medical reasons, such as the prevention of a nutrient deficiency or to help with the treatment of disease.[4] Examples of early diet therapy are the Sippy diet that used milk and cream to treat ulcers and the Kempner rice diet to treat hypertension; each was named for the physician who designed it.

As the dietitian's role in the hospital became one of providing specialized care and modifying diets to treat various medical conditions, the title, *clinical dietitian*, replaced the former titles.

In the early 1970s, reports of widespread malnutrition among hospitalized patients helped to increase the visibility of clinical dietitians.[5] Clinical dietitians began to take a more active role in screening and monitoring patients along with the provision of nutrition support. Development of individual nutrition care plans became important functions of clinical dietitians. As the role of diet in the etiology of chronic diseases became better defined, clinical dietitians began to spend a greater percentage of their time participating in the prevention of diseases such as heart disease, cancer, and diabetes.

EMPLOYMENT SETTINGS OF CLINICAL DIETITIANS

In the 2011 survey of registered dietitians (RDs) and dietetic technicians, registered (DTRs), 86 percent of those contacted reported they were currently employed in dietetics.[6] This high percentage of dietitians and dietetic technicians who were working in the field of dietetics reflected the diversity of job opportunities. **Tables 6-1, 6-2**, and **6-3** show the primary employment areas of dietitians. Fifty-six percent of RDs and 58 percent of DTRs were employed in clinical areas of practice. These findings and earlier membership surveys with similar findings indicate stability in these employment areas and that clinical areas of practice are the chosen area by entry-level professionals.

The primary areas of clinical practice are:

1. Acute care/inpatient
   Hospitals
2. Ambulatory care
   a. hospital outpatient departments
   b. clinics
   c. outpatient care centers

Table 6-1. Primary Practice Area of Dietitians

	RDs (%)	DTRs (%)
Clinical nutrition—acute care/inpatient	30	43
Clinical nutrition—ambulatory care	17	0
Clinical nutrition—long term care	9	15
Community nutrition	11	12
Food and nutrition management	12	18
Consultation and business	8	2
Education and research	7	2

Base: 8853 RDs and DTRs.
Source: Reprinted from Journal of the Academy of Nutrition and Dietetics, Volume 112, Number 1 (January 2012), Ward. B. "Compensation and Benefits Survey 2011, Moderate Growth in Registered Dietitian and Dietetic Technician, Registered, Compensation in the Past 2 years," 29–40, Copyright 2012, with permission from Elsevier.

3. Long-term care
   a. nursing homes
   b. assisted living facilities
   c. Alzheimer's disease units

Table 6-2. Highest Incidence Positions—RDs

	RDs (%)
Clinical dietitian	15
Outpatient dietitian, general	4
Outpatient dietitian, specialist—diabetes	4
Outpatient dietitian, specialist—renal	4
Clinical dietitian, long-term care	9
Women, infants, and children nutritionist	6
Director of food and nutrition services	4

Source: Reprinted from Journal of the Academy of Nutrition and Dietetics, Volume 112, Number 1 (January 2012), Ward. B. "Compensation and Benefits Survey 2011, Moderate Growth in Registered Dietitian and Dietetic Technician, Registered, Compensation in the Past 2 years," 29–40, Copyright 2012, with permission from Elsevier.

Table 6-3. Highest Incidence Positions—DTRs

	DTR
Dietetic technician, clinical	41
Clinical dietitian, long-term care	3
Dietetic technician, long-term care	12
WIC nutritionist	9
Director of food and nutrition service	6
Food service management	8

Source: Reprinted from Journal of the Academy of Nutrition and Dietetics, Volume 112, Number 1 (January 2012), Ward. B. "Compensation and Benefits Survey 2011, Moderate Growth in Registered Dietitian and Dietetic Technician, Registered, Compensation in the Past 2 years," 29–40, Copyright 2012, with permission from Elsevier.

PRACTICE AUDIT ACTIVITIES

In the 2010 Commission on Dietetic Registration Practice audit, the practice areas of RDs and DTRs were compared to show where there was a higher level of involvement. In clinical practice, the particular areas in which RDs had a higher level of involvement than DTRs included the following[7]:

- Principles of education including designing courses and evaluating education programs.
- Conducting research. Designing, developing proposals, reporting at professional conferences, and writing for publication.
- Providing nutrition care to individuals. This comprised the largest area of activity as would be expected and included development of institutional standards for nutrition care, evaluating clients' overall health status, recommending and writing orders for tube feedings, parenteral nutrition, medications, etc.
- Providing nutrition programs for population groups, which included designing services to meet nutrition-related needs of groups.

ORGANIZATION OF CLINICAL NUTRITION SERVICES

Clinical nutrition services may be organized in several ways, depending on the setting. In most hospitals, clinical nutrition services are managed by the director of clinical nutrition, or the chief clinical dietitian (**Figure 6-1a**). Typically, the chief clinical dietitian reports to an individual whose primary responsibilities are food service and the financial management of the entire food and nutrition department. In some instances, clinical dietetics may be organized as a separate department that reports to an executive or administrator with other patient care responsibilities such as nursing or pharmacy (**Figure 6-1b**). There are advantages and disadvantages to both types of organization. Combining clinical nutrition with food services can facilitate communication regarding patient food choices and menus. By contrast, having clinical nutrition as a separate department may increase visibility as an important patient care service unit distinct from food service.

a. The Methodist Hospital Food and Nutrition Services Organizational Chart 2012

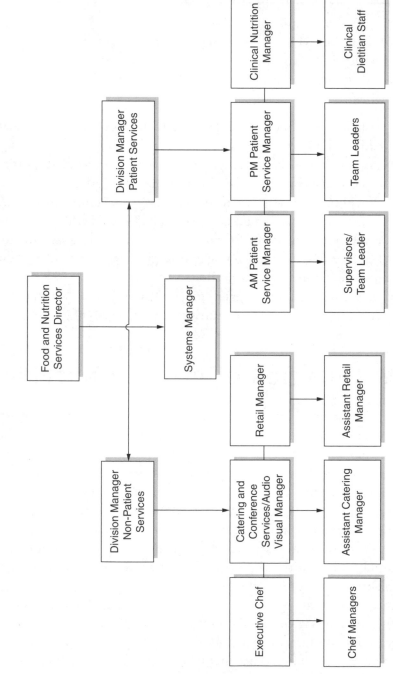

FIGURE 6-1. (*Continued*)

b. Clinical Nutrition Within a Separate Department

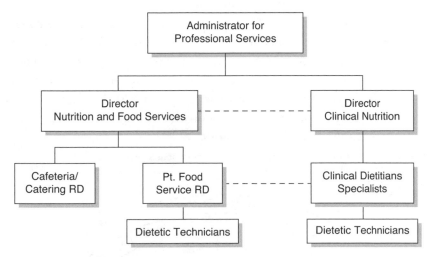

FIGURE 6-1a AND b. Examples of Nutrition and Food Service Organizational Charts.

Sources: Example a, ©2012 The Methodist Hospital, Houston, Texas. Example b is courtesy of Nutrition Center, Arkansas Children's Hospital, Little Rock, Arkansas.

RESPONSIBILITIES IN CLINICAL DIETETICS

Nutrition Care Process and Model

The Quality Management Committee of the Academy of Nutrition and Dietetics developed a nutrition care process (NCP) and model that was adopted by the house of delegates of the American Dietetic Association in 2003.[8] The purpose of the planning model was "for implementation and dissemination to the dietetics profession and the association for the enhancement of the practice of dietetics."[9] The NCP is defined as systematic problem-solving methods that dietetic professionals use to critically think and make decisions to address nutrition-related problems and to provide safe and effective quality nutrition care.

In 2008, a review and update of the process was undertaken following a survey of ADA groups experienced in using the NCP.[10] The process, now referred to as the nutrition care process and model (NCPM), included revisions in the original model and defined the functions under each step as follows (**Figure 6-2**):

1. *Nutrition assessment.* In step 1, a systematic approach to collect, record, and interpret relevant data from patients, clients, family members, caregivers, and other individual groups is undertaken. Examples of the type of data collected are food and nutrition-related history, anthropometric measurements, biochemical data, medical tests and procedures, nutrition-focused physical examination findings, and client history.

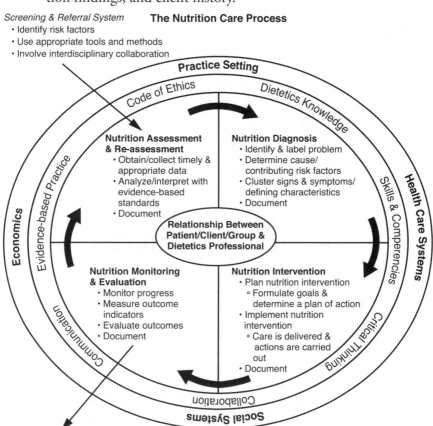

FIGURE 6-2. The Nutrition Care Process and Model.

Source: Reprinted from Journal of the American Dietetic Association 108, no. 7 (July 2008), "Nutrition Care Process and Model," 1116, 2008, with permission from Elsevier.

2. *Nutrition diagnosis.* Nutrition professionals identify and label existing nutrition problems they are responsible for treating independently. The determination for continuation of care follows this step.
3. *Nutrition intervention.* Action is taken with the intent of changing a nutrition-related behavior, risk factor, environmental condition, or aspect of health status. This entails writing a plan of care, collaborating with the patient or client to identify goals of the interaction, and partnering with the patient and other caregivers to carry out the plan.
4. *Nutrition monitoring and evaluation.* In this final step, the amount of progress is identified and whether the goals and expected outcomes are being met is determined. Three steps are involved:
   a. Monitor progress
   b. Measure the outcomes
   c. Evaluate the outcomes by comparing to earlier status or reference standards.

A standardized language or set of terms has been developed to describe the results in each step of the NCPM.[11] The terms are from the international dietetics and nutrition terminology (IDNT) to facilitate the inclusion of RD activities in electronic health record keeping, and also in policies, procedures, rules, and legislation. The use of such standardized reporting primarily assists in documenting nutrition care in the medical record in a way that will refer to each of the four steps in the NCPM and highlight the role of nutrition in patient care.

Medical Nutrition Therapy

Medical nutrition therapy (MNT) has been defined as "all diagnostic, therapeutic, or counseling services provided by an RD for management or treatment of any disease, condition, disorder, or illness."[12] A history of the development of MNT, its importance in the national healthcare discussion, and the challenges presented to members were discussed by the government relations office of the ADA in 2005.[13] Established by legislation under Medicare Part B, provision was made for Medicare reimbursement to dietitians for care in two disease conditions—diabetes and renal disease. The stipulation was that Medicare MNT providers must use evidence-based protocols or guides for practice to illustrate that the

MNT offered by RDs has a positive medical impact on patients and a positive impact on healthcare budgets. The rationale and justification for the successful passage of legislation extending MNT to other disease treatments depends, in large part, on the evidence that can be demonstrated regarding its beneficial effects. Cost containment is a critical part of all healthcare reform measures, and passage of any new MNT therapies will demand good scientific evidence of both its cost-effectiveness and efficacy. To this end, evidence-based outcomes research that documents the clinical effectiveness of MNT is all important. Evidence-based practice (EBP), it follows, improves the quality of care and helps manage costs. By adopting EBP in providing MNT, RDs will use the best available evidence to provide therapy, in addition to their own clinical expertise and experience.

The academy assists dietitians by maintaining a library of resources, the Evidence Analysis Library (EAL), available online at www.adaevidencelibrary .com. The EAL gathers the best, most current, and most relevant research on important questions in dietetic practice and is available at no cost to all ADA members.[14] The EAL offers evidence-based nutrition practice guidelines in areas such as lipid metabolism, adult weight management, and critical illnesses.

It can be noted that MNT describes the broad area of practice formerly called diet therapy or therapeutic dietetics, and NCPM is the application of nutrition therapies to disease conditions including guides for nutrition education and preventive nutrition care services.

Standards of Practice

The *Standards of Practice in nutrition care* describe the minimum expectations for competent nutrition care practice. The *Standards of Professional Performance*, a companion document, describe the expectation for competent behavior in the nondirect patient or client nutrition care aspect of RD and DTR roles. First developed in 2005, the standards were updated in 2008.[15]

The standards of practice (SOP) in nutrition care do the following:

- Address activities related to patient/client care during the NCP.
- Apply to RDs and DTRs who have direct contact with individual patient/client care in acute and long-term care, as well as in public health, community, extended care, and ambulatory care settings.

- Are formatted according to the four steps of the NCP (i.e., nutrition assessment, nutrition diagnosis, nutrition intervention, and nutrition monitoring and evaluation).
- Reflect the individual levels (RD and DTR) of training, responsibility, and accountability.

The standards of professional performance (SOPP) do the following:

- Address behaviors related to the professional role that are not in the NCP.
- Apply to RDs and DTRs in all practice settings.
- Address six domains of professional performance (i.e., provision of services, application of research, communication and application of knowledge, use and management of resources, quality in practice, and competence and accountability.
- Reflect the individual levels (RD and DTR) of training, responsibility, and accountability.

Standards of practice and standards of professional performance have also been developed by the academy in diabetes care, oncology, nutrition support, and behavioral health care.

THE CLINICAL NUTRITION SERVICE TEAM

Clinical nutrition services may be provided by a number of team members in healthcare facilities. Inpatient nutritional care in hospitals is usually the responsibility of persons in several positions—clinical nutrition managers or chief clinical dietitians, clinical dietitians, dietetic technicians, and dietetic assistants. Outpatient clinics and ambulatory care centers may use all four positions but are more likely to employ only clinical dietitians. Extended care facilities and physician offices may have clinical dietitians on staff; however, more often these facilities use a consulting dietitian to provide MNT for selected patients and clients. Consulting dietitians may be in private practice or part of a group practice.

Clinical Nutrition Manager or Chief Clinical Dietitian

The clinical nutrition manager or chief clinical dietitian is primarily responsible for directing the activities of clinical dietitians, dietetic technicians, and dietetic assistants. Major tasks performed include developing and managing budgets for the clinical area, hiring clinical nutrition employees, evaluating employee job performance, providing in-service and on-the-job training, reviewing productivity reports, writing job descriptions, scheduling employees, developing policies and procedures, designing performance standards, and developing and implementing goals and objectives for the department. The clinical nutrition manager is also responsible for communicating with the staff of other departments and the administration. Ultimately, the clinical nutrition manager ensures that performance is actually accomplished to achieve the goals and objectives for the department. The Clinical Nutrition Management dietetic practice group provides a newsletter and a yearly workshop on practice updates and opportunities for networking with peers.

Clinical Dietitian

The primary responsibility of the clinical dietitian is to provide nutritional care for patients. Clinical dietitians in hospitals are involved in nutritional screening for patients to determine the presence of or risk of developing malnutrition, to perform nutritional assessments, and to develop nutrition care plans. Clinical nutrition services may be provided to general patient-care units or may be based on a medical specialization (e.g., critical care or diabetes education). Clinical dietitians are important members of the healthcare team because they consult and collaborate with physicians, pharmacists, nurses, social workers, chaplains, and others in providing nutritional care.

Clinical dietitians are the source of authoritative knowledge about MNT and patient nutrition education. They routinely communicate with other disciplines regarding developments in MNT and patient education through in-service teams, rounds, and multidisciplinary patient care conferences.

Successful clinical dietitians in acute healthcare facilities must also be able to apply managerial concepts to provide effective nutritional care. Management tasks often performed by clinical dietitians include scheduling of patient care services, in-service training, on-the-job training, employee interviews and evaluations, writing, job descriptions, planning cycle menus, and evaluating the quality of patient food.

Typical activities of a clinical dietitian include the following[16]:

- Use the nutrition care process to screen, assess, diagnose, interview, and evaluate nutritional care of patients.
- Provide instruction to patients and families on nutritional needs.

- Review medical records for information including nutrition-related data.
- Calculate nutrient and fluid requirements.
- Evaluate nutrient intake and make adjustments accordingly.
- Adapt regular diets to meet individual needs or preferences.
- Plan oral diets with multiple nutritional requirements.
- Refer clients to community resources for ongoing service (Women, Infants, and Children program; Mobile Meals, outpatient clinics, wellness centers).
- Use evidence analysis in making practical decisions about needed care.
- Perform quality assurance and make performance improvements as needed.
- Utilize technology as freely as possible.
- Communicate with physicians, nurses, and other staff.
- Attend medical rounds.
- Provide ongoing evaluation for employees.
- Utilize SOP and SOPP in providing care.
- Serve as preceptor for dietetic interns and other students.

Clinical dietitians may be members of one or more dietetic practice groups. Besides working in general clinical practice, dietitians may be titled gerontological nutritionists, dietitians in developmental and psychiatric disorders, oncology dietitians, renal dietitians, pediatric dietitians, diabetes care and support, dietitians in nutrition support, perinatal nutritionists, and others. The diversity of specialty and subspecialty areas of practice reflects the broad range of interests and opportunities open to the clinical dietitian.

Dietetic Technician

The dietetic technician in the clinical setting assists the clinical dietitian and is a valuable member of the nutrition care team. Typically, major functions performed include gathering data for nutritional screening and assigning a level of risk for malnutrition according to predetermined criteria. He or she may help with nutritional assessments by gathering laboratory and anthropometric data, collecting and analyzing nutritional intakes, obtaining nutritional histories, and reviewing medical histories. Dietetic technicians may administer nourishment and dietary supplements for patients and monitor and document intakes. They may provide information to help patients select menus and give simple diet instructions.

Dietetic technicians maintain a high level of knowledge of nutritional care. Management responsibilities of dietetic technicians may also include supervision of dietetic assistants and students.

Dietetic Assistant

The dietetic assistant helps the clinical dietitian and dietetic technician in some of the routine aspects of nutritional care. He or she is often responsible for processing diet orders, checking patient intakes, giving nourishments, and transmitting special food requests. Dietetic assistants may also help distribute and pick up inpatient menus and pass and collect trays. They may be involved in evaluating food acceptance and gathering food records to evaluate and document nutrient intakes.

CLINICAL DIETETICS OUTLOOK

Healthcare Reform

Changes in healthcare are occurring at both local and national levels. Bills have been introduced in Congress at times aimed toward reforms of the healthcare system to provide affordable health care for everyone and to take cost-containment measures. The ADA/academy has lobbied for the inclusion of nutrition care expansion of MNT at every opportunity and continues to do so. The role of the clinical dietitian will expand as disease conditions beyond diabetes and renal disease, such as cardiovascular disease, obesity, and others, are allowed for reimbursement of services rendered by the RD.

Nutrition-related provisions of the Health Care Education and Reconciliation Act of 2010 are outlined in a recent issue of the *Academy of Nutrition and Dietetics Journal*, along with an outline of resources available to assist dietitians in undertaking healthcare reform.[17] While healthcare reform is expected to increase the need for food and nutrition services, it is less clear as to whether dietetics practitioners will be the only ones that provide the services. Potential areas for clinical dietitians to practice are in the new areas of primary care for both adults and children and in the "medical homes" for patients (especially those with chronic diseases). Nutrition care will become even more important in the preventive measures of the law. Clinical dietitians are in a unique position to make their voices heard, both in advocacy for inclusion in legislation implementing reforms and also in demonstrating their expertise in providing the highest quality nutritional care that is also cost effective.

Communicating Health Messages

As health care continues to expand beyond the traditional hospital and doctor's office settings, newer methods to reach the public are also being used. Telemedicine and telehealth care are being conducted via television to provide medical information. Programs by distance may be interactive, offering information exchange, or noninteractive, where information is transmitted but the recipients do not respond. Dietitians increasingly may be participants in such programs to transmit nutrition information in disease conditions. Busey and Michael point out both opportunities and pitfalls in such programs that may impact dietitians as they participate.[18] Electronic charting is another process that more hospitals are turning to, and this means that the clinical dietitians will need to be knowledgeable about this procedure and be prepared to fully implement it in practice. In the area of electronic charting of patient nutritional data, clinical dietitians and clinical managers must take the lead in order to provide the medical nutrition therapy needed.

The growth of online education in colleges and universities means students will be skilled in the use of technology as they enter practice. Through continuing education for professionals, dietitians may become technology proficient, if not already so. Consultation with patients and clients can be speeded up and made client oriented by helping them become more proactive in discovering and tracking information available on the Web. A virtual world appears to be on the horizon—a trend that dietitians can embrace to enhance their practice and make even greater contributions to health care.

Clinical Privileging

Clinical privileging refers to a process by which a hospital, specifically the governing body and the medical staff of the hospital, develop and implement procedures to ensure safe and quality patient care.[19,20] In most hospitals, the physician is the person responsible for overall patient care and assumes the risk and legal responsibility for the care, including prescribing diet orders. The dietetics profession has long discussed the possibility of the dietitian writing the diet order and ordering certain tests based on his or her certification, training, and experience.[21] Referred to as prescriptive authority, this can only occur if the RD demonstrates competence in advanced-level skills, is licensed by the state, and has specifically been approved by the hospital for this role. The dietitian must understand that certain legal responsibilities are assumed and that adherence to the scope of dietetic practice is a personal responsibility that will be periodically reviewed by the hospital and the medical staff.[22] Both federal and state regulations apply in the process of clinical privileging; however, as clinical dietitians attain advanced-level training and demonstrate competence and ability, more dietitians will assume this responsibility. In addition, compliance with the academy's code of ethics is required and will be monitored more closely in the future.[23] It should be noted in the earlier CDR audit of practice, some dietitians already have this responsibility and the practice is likely to grow.

Trends in Clinical Dietetics

Demographic trends have an impact on dietetic practice. For instance, the aging population and especially the growth of the oldest old means that nutrition is critical to helping keep this group healthy as long as possible. This is also the group that is at highest risk for chronic diseases that are treated in part with medical nutrition therapy. Increasing diversity among groups served has implications for dietitians in creating cultural competency and raising awareness.[24]

The obesity/overweight epidemic today is an area in which nutrition education for the public is more important than ever. Dietitians may find increasing opportunities to work with food processors, grocery stores, and advertisers to reach the public with the most effective nutrition messages. All these areas are discussed in more detail later in this text.

SUMMARY

Clinical dietetics is the largest area of employment for dietitians, especially at the entry level. Future roles will expand as new skills and competencies through advanced training and education are attained. Employment opportunities exist in acute care centers, in community-based programs, in consultation and private practice, in communications, and in many entrepreneurial undertakings.

The clinical dietitian is central in helping persons during illness through nutrition interventions. Equally important is helping individuals prevent the onset of chronic disease by the application of optimal nutrition practices throughout life. The expansion of MNT with cost-effectiveness data and demonstration of quality practice is a continuing challenge for the dietetics profession. Even though employment increasingly moves outside the traditional hospital or clinic, the services provided by the clinical dietitians will remain vital to the health and well-being of people experiencing illness and who need nutritional care.

DEFINITIONS

Clinical dietetics. The area of practice in which persons with illness or injury involving nutritional factors are treated using assessment, planning, and implementing nutrition care plans.

Clinical nutrition services. Activities provided in the practice of clinical dietetics, such as medical nutrition therapy and counseling.

Diet therapy. Treatment by diet; a term now replaced by *clinical nutrition therapy* or *medical nutrition therapy.*

Extended care facility. An institution that extends health care beyond the acute care setting when long-term term care is needed.

Medical nutrition therapy. The application of nutrition in the management of illness or injury.

Outpatient clinic. Treatment area of a hospital or healthcare facility in which patients are treated on an outpatient basis.

REFERENCES

1. Escott-Stump, S.A. "Our Nutrition Literacy Challenge: Making the 2010 Dietary Guidelines Relevant for Consumers." *Acad Nutr Diet J* 111 (2011);979.
2. Cooper, L.F. "The Dietitian and Her Profession." *J Am Diet Assoc* 14 (1938): 751–758.
3. See Note 2, p.752.
4. Huyck, L., and M.M. Rowe. "Managing Clinical Nutrition Services." (Rockville, MD: Aspen Publisher, 1990), 243.
5. Butterworth, E. "The Skeleton in the Hospital Closet." *Nutrition Today* 4 (1974): 4.
6. Ward, B. "Compensation and Benefits Survey 2011: Moderate Growth in Registered Dietitian and Dietetic Technician, Registered, Compensation in the Past 2 Years." *Acad Nutr Diet J* 112 (2012): 29–40.
7. Ward, B., D. Rogers, C. Mueller, R. Touger-Decker, K. L. Sauer, and D. Schmidt. "Distinguishing Entry-Level RD and DTR Practice: Results from the 2010 Commission on Dietetic Registration Entry-Level Dietetics Practice Audit." *J Am Diet Assoc* 111 (2011): 1749–1755.
8. Lacy, K., and E. Pritchett. "Nutrition Care Process and Model: ADA Adopts Road Map to Quality Care and Outcomes Management." *J Am Diet Assoc* 103 (2003): 1061–1071.

9. See Note 8.

10. Writing Group of the Nutrition Care Process/Standardized Language Committee. *J Am Diet Assoc* 108 (2008): 1113–1117.

11. Writing Group of the Nutrition Care Process and Standardized Language Committee. "Nutrition Care Process and Model Part II: Using the International Dietetics and Nutrition Terminology to Document the Nutrition Care Process." *J Am Diet Assoc* 9108 (2008): 1287–1293.

12. Smith, R.E., S. Patrick, P. Michael, and M. Hager. "Medical Nutrition Therapy: The Case of ADA's Advocacy Efforts (Part 1)." *J Am Diet Assoc* 105 (2005): 825–834.

13. Smith, R.E., S. Patrick, P. Michael, and M. Hager. "Medical Nutrition Therapy: The Case of ADA's Advocacy Efforts. (Part II)." *J Am Diet Assoc* 105 (2005): 987–996.

14. Blumberg-Kason, S., and R. Lipscomb. "Evidence-Based Nutrition Practice Guidelines: A Valuable Resource in the Evidence-Analysis Library." *J Am Diet Assoc* 106 (2006): 1935–1936.

15. American Dietetic Association Quality Management Committee. "American Dietetic Association Revised 2008 Standards of Practice for Registered Dietitians in Nutrition Care; Standards of Professional Performance for Registered Dietitians; Standards of Practice for Dietetic Technicians, Registered, in Nutrition Care; and Standards of Professional Performance for Dietetic Technician, Registered." *J Am Diet Assoc* 108 (2008): 1538–1543.

16. Ward, B., C. Mueller, R. Touger-Decker, and K.L. Sauer. "Entry-Level Dietetics Practice Today: Results from the 2010 Commission on Dietetic Registration Entry-Level Dietetics Practice Audit." *J Am Diet Assoc* 111 (2011): 914–941.

17. Turner, P.A. "An Overview of the Intentions of Health Care Reform." *Acad Nutr Diet J* 112, suppl. 1 (2012): S56–S63.

18. Busey, J.C., and P. Michael. "Telehealth—Opportunities and Pitfalls." *J Am Diet Assoc* 108 (2008): 1296–1301.

19. Hager, M.H. "Clinical Privileging for Registered Dietitians. A Regulatory Perspective." *J Am Diet Assoc* 107 (2007): 558–560.

20. Hager, M.H., and S.M. McCauley. "Clinical Privileging: What It Is—and Isn't." *J Am Diet Assoc* 109 (2009): 400–402.

21. See Note 18.

22. Weil, S.D., L. Lafferty, K.S. Keim, D. Sowa, and R. Dowling. "Registered Dietitian Prescriptive Practices in Hospitals." *J Am Diet Assoc* 108 (2008): 1688–1692.

23. ADA. "American Dietetic Association Commission on Dietetic Registration Code of Ethics for the Profession of Dietetics and Process for Consideration of Ethics Issues." *J Am Diet Assoc* 109 (2009): 1461–1467.

24. Rhea, M. "Future Change Driving Dietetic Workforce Supply and Demand; Future Scan. 2012–2022." *Acad Nutr Diet J* suppl. 1 (2012): S10–S24.

CHAPTER 7

Management in Food and Nutrition Systems

"Food management RDs need to have technical expertise, knowledge, and interpersonal skills."[1]

OUTLINE

INTRODUCTION

Food and food service are prominent in the history of the profession of dietetics. One of the main purposes of the first organized meeting of the American Dietetic Association was to discuss ways of meeting food shortages during World War I. Many of the first members of the association served overseas feeding hospitalized soldiers and people living under wartime conditions. Cooking schools, scientists who produced the first tables of food values, early day soup kitchens, and school lunch programs were among the forerunners of institutions that fed the public.[2]

Food service in hospitals was the primary focus of the first dietitians. During the 1890s, food service in hospitals was managed by the chef, the housekeeper, or the nursing department. In the early 1900s, however, many dietitians were in charge of dietary departments and had the responsibility for all food service as well as teaching nurses and providing diet therapy for patients with metabolic diseases. Hospital dietitians dealt with budgets, department organization, personnel management, and quality food service. Nutrition was recognized as an aspect of medicine, and food prescriptions were handled as apothecary compounds, thus creating a demand for special diet kitchens. The hospital dietitian had the same status as the superintendent of nurses and was recognized as the nutrition expert.[3]

Dietitians with food service management responsibilities became members of the Food Administration section in the ADA, and their practice was referred to as *administrative dietetics*. The terminology now used is *management in food and nutrition systems*.

Management is discussed fully later in the text as a skill needed by dietitians in all areas of practice.

ACTIVITIES OF ENTRY-LEVEL DIETITIANS AND DIETETIC TECHNICIANS

In 2010, the Commission on Dietetic Registration conducted a practice audit among dietitians and dietetic technicians and indicated the percentage of time spent in selected activities. Management activities of both groups are shown in **Table 7-1**.

Table 7-1. Management Activities of Entry-Level Dietitians and Dietetic Technicians

Activity (Percent)	RD	DTR*
Managing human resources		
Assign or schedule staff	15	25
Make decisions on personnel actions	10	23
Comply with labor relations	15	23
Evaluate performance of staff	22	31
Managing food and material resources		
Maintain safety and sanitation of food, facilities, or equipment	27	53
Monitor storage conditions	22	39
Develop menus for clients with normal needs	33	45
Evaluate food products by taste, smell, and appearance	33	50
Calculate quantities to purchase of food other material resources	9	21
Purchase food, nutritional supplements, equipment, or supplies	14	24
Assess client satisfaction with food and/or nutrition service	40	59
Adjust daily menu, food production, or distribution based on availability of food, labor, or equipment	11	30
Institute or maintain sustainability practices	8	18
Manage facilities		
Maintain facilities and equipment	11	24
Assure safety of employees, patients, clients, and customers	25	38

*The higher percentages of involvement by dietetic technicians in many of the management categories reflect the areas in which technicians are most often employed. This was a survey of entry-level professionals, and it should be noted that more dietitians begin their careers in clinical areas of practice; this was borne out in those particular areas surveyed.

Notes: RD = registered dietitian; DTR = dietetic technician, registered.

Source: Reprinted from Journal of the American Dietetic Association 111, Number 11 (November 2011), Ward, B., D. Rogers, C. Mueller, R. Touger-Decker, KI.L. Sauer, C. Schmidt, "Distinguishing Entry-Level RD and DTR Practice: Results from the 2010 Commission on Dietetic Registration Entry-Level Dietetics Practice Audit, 1749–1755, Copyright 2011, with permission from Elsevier.

AREAS OF EMPLOYMENT

In the 2011 membership survey, 12 percent of registered dietitians (RDs) and 18 percent of dietetic technicians, registered (DTRs) indicated their practice is in food and nutrition management. Further, 22 percent of practitioners are executives, directors, or managers, and another 19 percent are supervisors or coordinators. The results were similar among both RDs and DTRs.[4]

In the same study, it was reported that salaries for the food and nutrition manager are the highest of those in any practice area. The salaries reflect both geographic location and years of experience as the food and nutrition manager is nearly always a dietitian with work experience beyond entry level and may have an advanced degree or a business degree.

Dietitians in food and nutrition management typically affiliate with one or more of the following four dietetic practice groups: Management in Food and Nutrition Systems, Dietitians in Business and Communication, School Nutrition Services, and Food and Culinary Professionals. In addition, clinical managers may belong to the Clinical Nutrition Management group. Dietitians in food and nutrition management may be identified through a wide range of titles, such as coordinator, specialist, executive dietitian, director of food and nutrition services, director of clinical nutrition, or chief administrator.

Practice areas are often categorized by work settings, such as food and nutrition management in acute care, long-term care, and noninstitutional employment areas. To encompass the broader management area, clinical nutrition management, commercial food service, and school nutrition are added to this list. A discussion of each follows.

Food and Nutrition Management in Acute Care

Food service in acute care is the type of service provided in hospitals or similar healthcare institutions in which patients receive short-term medical treatment, usually 1–5 days. Several characteristics of this type of food service are:

1. Fast turnover of patients with day-to-day fluctuations in the number of meals prepared and served.
2. Special diets requiring different types of food preparation. In some instances, as many as 50 percent of all patients will require special or modified diets.

3. Selective menus for patients, increasing the number of food items prepared.
4. Multiple serving systems in an institution, such as individual tray service, decentralized service with pantries on patient floors, and restaurant-style service providing individualized patient service.

In some institutions, food is prepared in bulk, then preportioned and held until the time of meal service, when it is rethermalized and served. In others, food is prepared centrally just before meal service and either portioned individually or sent in bulk to patient areas for individual service. Production and food service systems vary, but in each system, the dietitian has overall responsibility for food production and service or may share this responsibility with a dietetic technician, chef, or manager. Whatever the scope of his or her responsibility, the dietitian must be knowledgeable in food production techniques, food purchasing, safety and sanitation, strategic planning, human relations, communication skills, managerial skills, and financial management.

Food and Nutrition Management in Long-Term Care Facilities

The provision of food for clients in nursing homes, extended care facilities, and correctional institutions is included in the long-term care category. Food service in these institutions differs from that in acute care in that clients are long term and are usually served in group settings. Central food production and few special diets are typical because most of the long-term clients will be following a normal, healthy eating pattern. The food service, especially in smaller nursing homes and extended care facilities, may be managed by a dietetic technician or by a certified dietary manager under the direction of a dietitian consultant. In correctional institutions, the day-to-day management is often provided by nonprofessionals under the direction of a dietitian consultant when one is available. All aspects of food service management are equally as important in long-term care as in the hospital with the added necessity of ensuring nutritional adequacy and acceptability over longer periods of time. In almost all long-term facilities, there are federal and state regulations relating to the provision of food services to clients that must be followed for the institution to receive government funding and provide quality care. The qualifications for the food service manager are also specified in the regulations.

Food and Nutrition Management in Noninstitutional Settings

Management of food and nutrition in noninstitutional settings is typically provided in colleges and universities, employee cafeterias, and business and commercial enterprises. The food service may be for-profit or non-profit, depending on the type of institution. Generally, institutions serving the public will be for profit while schools or businesses providing employee food services are more often nonprofit. Clients choose to patronize the food services offered and the type of food services may vary widely. A college or university, for instance, may offer cafeteria, dining room, restaurant, catering, and vending services. School and employee food service is often provided by cafeteria service along with vending and dining room service. Many businesses provide employee cafeterias or restaurant service. The dietitian's responsibility is to provide food that is safe and acceptable to the customers, meets financial expectations, and promotes good nutrition.

School Nutrition Programs

School nutrition programs, offering either lunch or breakfast, or both, are available in almost all public schools through grade 12.[5] In 2009, about 31 million students from preschool through grade 12 were fed daily.[6] An average of 11 million children per day participated in the federal school breakfast program in 2009. The programs are administered and partially funded by the federal government, and they must meet specific guidelines for nutritional quality of meals and for student eligibility. Free or reduced-price meals are provided based on the family economic status. The emphasis is on long-term health benefits for children through establishing good eating habits. The following is a position statement supporting school nutrition programs:

> It is the position of the American Dietetic Association, School Nutrition Association, and Society for Nutrition Education that comprehensive, integrated nutrition services in schools, kindergarten through grade 12, are an essential component of coordinated school health programs that will improve the nutritional status, health, and academic performance of our nation's children. Local school wellness policies may strengthen comprehensive nutrition services in schools by providing opportunities for multidisciplinary teams to identify and address local school needs.[7]

Dietitians in school nutrition programs need both managerial and nutrition education skills. That school nutrition programs provide satisfying careers to many is shown in a recent study of job satisfaction; dietitians with management responsibilities, including those in school child nutrition programs, showed the highest level of satisfaction with the nature of the work and a higher overall level of satisfaction compared to national indices.[8]

The customer is the most important consideration when offering school food service that meets strict guidelines for safety and nutritional quality while also controlling costs.[9] Some programs use websites to promote offerings and others use newspaper advertising to publish menus and gain public support.

Clinical Nutrition Management

As discussed earlier, the clinical nutrition manager is the professional who directs the activities of a clinical unit in hospitals and healthcare institutions. This may include responsibility for one or more units and the supervision of other professionals in clinical areas. The clinical manager performs many of the same management functions as the food service dietitian—management of human, financial, and material resources. The clinical dietitian who progresses from an entry-level position to a management position will normally have 5–10 years or more of experience and may not be involved in day-to-day activities directly related to patient care.

Commercial Food Service

Commercial food service is described as retail and hospitality food service establishments that prepare food for immediate consumption on or off premises. The types of establishments employing dietitians include independent restaurants, catering services, casual and family dining restaurants, and fine dining restaurants. Supermarket chains, limited service (fast-food) chains, and hotel chains also have high potential for dietetic services. Five specific areas of need in these institutions are nutrition education, healthful menu planning, recipe and menu analysis, marketing, and quality assurance.

Skills in public relations, communications, marketing, purchasing, and financial management are expected of dietitians who work in commercial food services. Therefore, additional training and experience are often needed by the dietitian to be fully qualified for these roles.

Additional Areas of Opportunity

Additional opportunities for dietitians in food service management include positions in food corporations, such as research and development, consumer affairs, communications, government liaison, emergency feeding for displaced persons, disaster planning centers, military-based homeless shelters and food distribution centers, worldwide religious ministries and government food programs, adult and child care programs; and academic units with food, nutrition, or hospitality programs. Many dietitians are employed in contract food service companies that provide for-profit management services. Hospitals, colleges and universities, schools, employee cafeterias in businesses, hotels and restaurants, and healthcare institutions may contract with a company who manages food services for a negotiated fee. The companies hire and often train their own personnel, including dietitian managers.

STANDARDS FOR PROFESSIONAL PERFORMANCE

In 2001, an Academy of Nutrition and Dietetics group developed standards for professional practices in management and food service settings—a first innovative step.[10] The standards described the minimum expectations in management and food service settings for quality service, the analysis of practices performed, and the services that maximize the nutritional health and well-being of clients or customers. The standards applied to the following areas of practice: application of research, communication, application of knowledge, utilization and management of resources, and quality in practice; the standards include the rationale, indicators, and examples of outcomes.

In 2009, *Standards of Practice and Standards of Professional Performance* replaced the earlier standards.[11] The standards describe a competent level of professionalism and the professional role behaviors that relate to quality of care and administrative practice, resource management, education, professional environment, ethics, collaboration, research, and resource allocation.[12] According to Puckett,[13] today's management RD must, at a minimum, possess competencies in the following areas:

- Environmental protection rules
- The political environment
- Marketing and customer satisfaction
- Continual quality improvement
- Work design and productivity
- Innovative cost-containment measures
- Food-consumption patterns
- Human resource trends
- Food and water safety

- Disaster and emergency planning
- Project and process management
- Cultural diversity in the marketplace

Characteristics of Successful Food and Nutrition Managers

Dietitians in food and nutrition management need to exhibit leadership qualities similar to those in all areas of business, healthcare institutions, schools, and other sites of practice. They must manage personnel and financial resources, produce quality products and services, and communicate effectively within the organization and to the larger community. A list of competencies needed by healthcare food service directors is shown in **Table 7-2**. The competencies are typical of visionary leaders who are effective in their position and in the organization.

Table 7-2. Competencies Needed by Healthcare Food Service Managers

Successful healthcare food service managers will:

- Use management techniques to cultivate relationships in and out of the institution and achieve cooperation through teamwork.
- Demonstrate effective communications to achieve understanding of personnel and departmental policies.
- Achieve an organizational structure, mission statement, policies, and procedures that effect necessary changes when indicated.
- Possess technological knowledge of food service, practice experience, and external business and administrative needs.
- Use management techniques based on sound character, compassion, insight, and personal integrity.
- Exhibit personal behaviors and attitudes consistent with professional and institutional goals.
- Pursue professional knowledge and growth.
- Possess effective supervisory and managerial skills to derive optimal employee performance.
- Achieve ways to enhance performance and growth of employees.
- Understand the policies of the institution and an ability to interface effectively with superiors.
- Exhibit effective use of resources (fiscal, personnel, and material) to facilitate planning and current operations.
- Possess analytic and decision-making techniques to achieve maximum quality for customers and clients.
- Formulate a creative vision that integrates mutually satisfying department and institutional goals.

Source: Adapted from Journal of the American Dietetic Association, 95, Watabe-Dawson, M. "Visionary Leaders are Key to Success in Food Service" p. 13. Copyright 1995, with permission from Elsevier.

Job Satisfaction Survey

A survey among RDs with management responsibilities was conducted at Kansas State University to explore the multiple facets of job satisfaction and intent to leave a position.[14] Members of three different dietetic practice groups were contacted. Nine facets of jobs were explored for satisfaction levels. The nature of the work received the highest rating, with supervision and coworkers also scoring high. Overall, every job facet scored higher than on an earlier job satisfaction survey that reported occupations of both public and private employers in the United States. Scores varied according to income level, budget responsibility, and the number of other RDs worked with, but overall, there was a high level of satisfaction and a low score for intent to leave.

EXPANDED OPPORTUNITIES

Entry-level dietitians with management responsibilities are employed primarily in food service or clinical nutrition service operations. The predominant responsibilities at this level involve technical skills that ensure that food is procured, managed, prepared, and delivered to patients and other clients, and that appropriate nutrition services are provided. With experience and perhaps advanced study, conceptual skills are utilized to identify problem areas requiring attention, to select appropriate techniques, to analyze alternative strategies, and to select solutions consistent with organization goals.

From entry-level positions, dietitians may advance to the assistant or associate director level of a department and eventually to director or chief administrator. They may manage multidepartmental units or a complex of smaller hospitals, specialty clinics, or long-term care centers. They may become the chief operating officer of a healthcare facility.

Dietitians directing food and nutrition services must have a diversified, multipurpose, broad-based education and experiences from which to draw for expanded roles. They must be familiar with applicable computer software, business organization, marketing, labor relations, industrial engineering, writing and media relations, public relations, financial management data evaluation, policy formation and problem solving, decision making, negotiation, behavior modification techniques, and dealing with challenges.

Expanded roles may include new and challenging positions that grow from the foundation the dietitian receives and that may not even generally be associated with dietetics. In health care, for instance, there is heightened consumer interest in what constitutes healthy food. The food industry wants effective marketing of its products, including information about safety and nutrient value, and it wants to develop new products. All these areas represent opportunities in consumer education, writing, food safety, media positions, public policy, food demonstration, and more.

SUMMARY

The dietitian in food service management has career opportunities in food, food production and service, management, and the higher levels of activities associated with management and leadership. For the motivated and skilled dietitians, higher salary levels and greater degrees of responsibility and self-actualization can be realized.

DEFINITIONS

Food production. The process of preparing and serving food, including purchasing, storage, and processing.

Food services. Production and service of food; also refers to the unit or group responsible for feeding groups.

Food service systems. Activities that together form the inputs, transformation, and outputs that make up an entire food operation.

Human resources. The personnel in an organization.

Management. The administration and coordination of the activities and functions in an organizational unit.

Quality assurance. The certification of the continual, optimal, effective, and efficient outcomes of a service or program.

Resource allocation. The equitable distribution of financial, physical, and human capital.

REFERENCES

1. Puckett, R.P., W. Barkley, G. Dixon, K. Egan, C. Koch, T. Malone, J. Scott-Smith, B. Sheridan, and M. Theis. "The American Dietetic Association Standards of Professional Performance for Registered Dietitians (Generalist and Advanced) in Management of Food and Nutrition Systems." *J Am Diet Assoc* 109 (2009): 540–543.
2. Cassell, J.A. *Carry the Flame: The History of the American Dietetic Association.* (Chicago: American Dietetic Association, 1990).

3. Barker, A., M. Foltz, M.B.F. Arensberg, and M.R. Schiller. *Leadership in Dietetics: Achieving a Vision for the Future.* (Chicago: American Dietetic Association, 1994).

4. Ward, B. "Compensation and Benefits Survey 2011: Moderate Growth in Registered Dietitian and Dietetic Technician, Registered, Compensation in the Past 2 Years." *Acad Nutr Diet J* 112 (2012): 29–40.

5. Story, M. "The Third School Nutrition Dietary Assessment Study: Findings and Policy Implications for Improving the Health of U.S. Citizens." *J Am Diet Assoc* 9109 (2009): S7–S13.

6. "Position of the American Dietetic Association, School Nutrition Association, and Society for Nutrition Education: Comprehensive School Nutrition Services." *J Am Diet Assoc* 110 (2010): 1738–1748.

7. See Note 6.

8. Sauer, K., D. Canter, and C. Shanklin. "Job Satisfaction of Dietitians with Management Responsibilities: An Exploratory Study Supporting ADA's Research Priorities." *J Am Diet Assoc* 110 (2010): 1432–1440.

9. Boyce, B. "Satisfying Customers and Lowering Costs in Foodservice: Can Both Be Accomplished Simultaneously?" *J Am Diet Assoc* 111 (2011): 1458–1466.

10. Griffin, B., J.M. Dunn, and I.F. Speranza. "Standards of Professional Practice for Dietetics Professionals in Management and Food Service Settings." *J Am Diet Assoc* 101 (2011): 944–946.

11. See Note 1.

12. See Note 1.

13. Puckett, R.P. "Leadership: Managing for Change." In *Food Service Manual for Health Care Institutions*, 3rd ed. (San Francisco: Jossey-Bass, 2004), p. 30–32.

14. See Note 8.

The Community Nutrition Dietitian

"Primary prevention is the most effective and affordable course of action for preventing and reducing the risk for chronic disease."[1]

OUTLINE

- Introduction
- Community Nutrition Practice
- Public Health Nutrition
  - Prevention
  - Levels of Prevention
- Activities of Community Dietitians
- Career Paths
  - Specialty Areas of Practice
- Career Outlook
- Summary
- Definitions
- References

INTRODUCTION

Community nutrition is the branch of nutrition that addresses the entire range of food and nutrition issues relating to individuals, families, and special groups with a common bond such as place of residence, language, culture, and health. Community nutrition programs include those that provide increased access to food resources, food and nutrition education, and health care. Public health nutrition is the component of community nutrition that is publicly funded and provided through a state or local health agency to promote health, prevent disease, and provide primary care. The community dietitian, community nutritionist, or public health nutritionist is the dietetic professional who provides nutrition services to identified groups.

Community nutrition professionals establish links with other professionals involved with the broad range of human services, including child care agencies, services to the elderly, educational institutions, and community-based research. They focus on promoting optimum health and preventing disease in the community by using a population and systems focus and a client or personal health service approach.[2]

Community health is influenced by the collective beliefs and practices of everyone in a community. It is estimated that 70 percent of all premature deaths in the United States are caused by environmental factors and individual behaviors.[3] The costs of health care for obesity and its complications, for instance, continue to rise as the incidence of this controllable condition rises among the American population. Childhood obesity is a particular risk as it often leads to adult obesity and chronic diseases later in life. Dietitians need to continue to demonstrate the value they bring to the economic burden of rising health costs that are estimated to be in the billions each year. Recent estimates of the healthcare costs related to obesity alone are over $190 billion per year, or approximately 21 percent of all healthcare expenditures, and this does not include the cost of lost productivity, poor quality of life, or accommodations that must be made in equipment, seating, etc.[4]

COMMUNITY NUTRITION PRACTICE

Community and public health dietitians work in many settings that focus on improving the health of a population group. Positions are characterized by an emphasis on health and wellness and the application of nutrition science to maintain health. Community dietitians often work in federal, state, or local public health agencies; neighborhood or community health centers; industry; ambulatory care clinics; home health agencies and specialized community projects; nonprofit and for-profit private and community health agencies/institutions; private practice and hospitals; and private and public schools.

Opportunities exist for community dietitians to participate in policy planning and implementation at federal, state, and local levels. A specific example is in the area of child care facilities. This is a growing industry as more and more infants and children are placed in day care, after-school care, and mother's day out programs, etc. The American Dietetic Association (ADA) published a position paper entitled *Benchmarks for Nutrition in Child Care.*[5] The position of the ADA, now called the Academy of Nutrition and Dietetics, states that "child care programs should achieve recommended benchmarks for meeting children's nutrition needs in a safe, sanitary, and supportive environment that promotes optimal growth and development."[6] Community dietitians are the most appropriate professionals to implement and monitor these benchmarks.

An example of ADA collaboration with other community professionals and organizations was in adopting a position paper, *Comprehensive School Nutrition Services.*[7] This joint position of the ADA, the School Nutrition Association, and the Society for Nutrition Education supports comprehensive integrated nutrition services in schools as an essential component of coordinated health programs. Community dietitians are active in this effort and many will be needed either on a part-time or full-time basis to fill the need in the near future.

The Academy of Nutrition and Dietetics has recently joined in a national initiative to end hunger and achieve food security,[8] an issue that community dietitians and public health nutritionists have long supported and worked towards. This collaboration includes community nutrition dietitians, health professionals, agricultural professionals, and food industry and hunger relief professionals. As food and nutrition experts, registered dietitians (RDs) can be at the forefront of solving the problems of hunger and food insecurity, which ironically also impacts obesity as well.

Every state has a department of health employing public health dietitians. Many states also use dietitians in programs such as Native American health service, health and human services or welfare, department of education (school nutrition programs), and in area agencies for the aging. The land-grant university in each state administers the cooperative extension program in which nutritionists, nutrition educators, and expanded food and nutrition educators are employed.

PUBLIC HEALTH NUTRITION

Practice in community nutrition focuses on the community as a whole and includes those activities that deal with groups rather than individuals. The largest subunit of community nutrition is public health nutrition. Whereas the practice area of community nutrition tends to be large and has a small body of defining literature, public health nutrition is well defined and includes a large body of literature discussing its role and defining characteristic. Public health dietitians tend to work in federal, state, or local agencies.

To understand what a public health dietitian does requires familiarity with the field of public health. All segments of the population, including the healthy and those who are vulnerable to or experiencing chronic disease, are targeted. Assessment of health needs, applying preventive measures, and intervening with treatments and rehabilitation are core functions. This epidemiologic approach is distinguished from the clinical approach, which more often concentrates on one-on-one assessment and care. Health promotion and disease prevention through service and research are requirements of all public health personnel.

The public health nutritionist establishes linkages with related community nutrition programs, nutrition education, food assistance, social or welfare services, care services to the elderly, other human services, and community-based research. The public health approach has the following characteristics[9]:

- Interventions that promote health and prevent communicable or chronic diseases by managing or controlling the community environment
- The promotion of a healthy lifestyle as a shared value for all people
- Directing money and energy to the problems that affect the lives of the largest number of people in the community
- Targeting the unserved or underserved by virtue of income, age, ethnicity, heredity, or lifestyle who are vulnerable to disease, hunger, or malnutrition
- Collaboration of the public, consumers, community leaders, legislators, policy makers, administrators, and health and human services professionals in assessing and responding to community needs and consumer demands
- Monitoring the health of the people in the community to ensure that the public health system achieves its objectives and responds to needs

Prevention

The prevention of illness is the primary purpose of public health. Prevention may take place at any point along the spectrum from prevention of disease to the prevention of impairment or disability. Prevention has three essential components: personal health, community-based, and social or system-based components. Each component has a distinct role, importance, and focus. Community nutrition practice involves making appropriate and coordinated use of each. Personal health deals with prevention issues at the individual level, such as working with a client to improve the diet for health promotion purposes. Community-based prevention uses campaigns that focus, for example, on increased consumption of fruits and vegetables or weight maintenance. Social policies focus on changing policies and laws such as those regarding food safety, tobacco, or alcohol so that the goals of prevention practice are achieved.

Levels of Prevention

For each of the three components of prevention, there are three levels of service.[10] Primary prevention includes healthcare services, medical tests, counseling, and health education, along with other actions designed to prevent a certain condition, such as education and counseling to reduce intakes of saturated fat and cholesterol to prevent cardiovascular disease. Secondary prevention includes measures such as healthcare services to identify or treat those who have an unknown disease or risk factors for a disease but are not yet experiencing symptoms of the disease. An example would be counseling persons with hypertension to prevent further complications. Tertiary prevention includes preventive healthcare measures of services that are part of the treatment and management of persons with clinical illnesses. Counseling for existing diseases and rehabilitation are examples of this type of health promotion.

ACTIVITIES OF COMMUNITY DIETITIANS

About 11 percent of RDs and 12 percent of dietetic technicians, registered (DTRs) work in community nutrition. The Special Supplemental Nutrition Program for Women, Infants, and Children (WIC) employs 6 percent of the RDs and 9 percent of the DTRs.[11]

Nutrition professionals in community nutrition need a general base of knowledge and a level of expertise in a chosen area (such as the needs of pregnant women, older persons, or migrant individuals). The ability to use scientific methods to study, interpret, promote, and apply findings to public health problems through a knowledge of research is essential to practice. Community nutrition professionals need to understand the nutritional needs across the life cycle, need to be able to use computer technology efficiently, and must be aware of multiethnic needs as community groups will generally be composed of several ethnic groups.[12] To be a credible nutrition resource, the RD must understand the fundamentals of nutrition, food science, and dietetics and have an underlying knowledge of human physiology, chemistry, biochemistry, and behavioral sciences. Changing behavior by providing information about foods that are affordable and available in local markets is a vital part of the counseling process.

In practice, dietitians in community programs are knowledgeable in and possess skills in several areas that include the following[13]:

- Assessment and prioritization of nutrition problems for various age and population groups using anthropometric, biochemical, clinical, dietary, and socioeconomic techniques
- Federal, regional, state, and local governmental structures and processes involved in the development of public policy, legislation, and regulations that influence and relate to nutrition and health services
- Political and ethical considerations within and across organizations and their impact on agency planning, policy, and decision making
- The integration of nutrition services into the overall health agency mission, goals, and plans
- Epidemiologic approaches to assessing the health and nutrition problems and trends in the community
- Monitoring, technical assistance, guidance, consultation, and collaboration within and across agencies and organizations
- Multidisciplinary and interdisciplinary team membership or leading
- Selection and/or development of nutrition education materials and approaches appropriate for individuals or small groups within the target population
- Media strategies used in print, broadcasting, and telecommunications, such as video and the Internet, to reach population groups

The dietitian's duties may include training of other agency staff as well as providing technical assistance to other professionals; serving as a resource to the public, media, business and industry; and advocating for needed nutrition policy at the local, state, and/or federal level. Other responsibilities may include advising the agency administrator, policy makers, and staff on current nutrition research that can contribute to the public's health and to the organization's mission, policies, and programs.

CAREER PATHS

As noted earlier, over half the dietitians employed in community nutrition work in the WIC program. WIC provides food, screening, and nutrition education and works to provide access to health services for low-income pregnant, breastfeeding, and nonbreastfeeding women and their children up to 5 years of age. It is administered by the U.S. Department of Agriculture, which provides funding to state agencies for the program. Other positions include those in maternal and child nutrition, adult health, food service management, children with special health needs, and programs in aging.

Another important area of practice is cooperative extension, administered through land-grant colleges and universities. The primary responsibilities in this area of practice include planning, developing, and implementing nutrition and health-related programs for all age groups in a county or district within a state, as well as developing a network of volunteers through adult and 4-H programs that further program goals. Other dietitians may work in corrections institutions and as home care dietitians.[14]

Specialty Areas of Practice

Several career paths are available to the public health nutritionist in areas considered specialties. Typical of these, and the knowledge needed, are the following:

- Adult health promotion or chronic disease prevention and control specialists may work in healthcare facilities, work-site health promotion, and community health agencies. Knowledge of nutritional management of specific chronic diseases and behavior and lifestyle change methodologies is required.
- Specialists working with healthcare needs related to developmental diseases and chronic disabling conditions need clinical knowledge of

child growth and development with an emphasis on the effects of mental retardation, developmental disabilities, and rehabilitation. Knowledge of techniques of feeding under special conditions is also required.

- Maternal and child health specialists understand principles of nutrition in pregnancy and lactation and in infancy, childhood, and adolescence. This includes the physical, psychological, and socioeconomic aspects of these early periods of life.

- Communications and media specialists must have knowledge of how individuals learn and of nutrition education methodology. They must also know how to use media effectively to design and implement nutrition promotion campaigns through a variety of communication channels, including television, radio, newspapers, magazines, and computers in various settings.

- Data management and nutrition surveillance nutritionists require additional training in biostatistics, epidemiology, informatics, and computer-based data management. Their responsibilities include the development of user-friendly systems for collecting, analyzing, interpreting, and presenting numerical data to be used in community program planning.

- Environmental health and food safety specialists have advanced knowledge and skills in food science, processing technology, microbiology, epidemiology, and food safety laws and regulations. They must be able to interpret federal, state, and local regulations regarding food safety.

- Food service systems managers for healthcare and group care facilities specialists have in-depth knowledge of food service systems management, healthcare financing, clinical nutrition, and nutritional care planning.

- Home health specialists have advanced knowledge of medical nutrition therapy for chronic disease and chronic disabling conditions of adults and children.

- Research specialists need to know how to prepare grant proposals, manage data, coordinate field-based studies, and design research protocols and analyze large data sets.

- Educators of public health nutrition professionals must have the knowledge and skills to prepare students for practice in public/community health.

CAREER OUTLOOK

Widespread health concerns exist today. The growing epidemic of obesity and its complications is a huge multifaceted problem with economic, social, and psychological implications. Food availability, food safety, health disparities among ethnic groups, nutrition information, and misinformation all impact public health. The community dietitian has an important role to play in helping meet these concerns. Involvement in policy decisions; obtaining advanced clinical skills; advanced study in epidemiology and research methodology; and extensive use of evidence-based research are examples of the ways dietitians can help meet critical community health needs. Dietitians who are prepared with managerial and conceptual skills as well as informatics will be increasingly needed in long-range program planning and policy implementation in communities.

SUMMARY

Community nutrition is an area in which professionals interact with community groups and individuals to promote health and prevent disease. Dietitians and nutritionists working in community nutrition hold positions in areas of public health; programs for the aging; cooperative extension; outpatient and public health clinics; federal, state and local governments; and agencies dealing with chronic disease. The emphasis is on meeting the nutritional needs of persons during all stages of life, thus maintaining health and preventing disease.

DEFINITIONS

Client. The recipient of services or products.
Community health. Health measures applied to groups of people.
Community nutrition. The branch of nutrition that addresses nutrition issues and services for groups of people.
Human health specialists. Nutrition professionals with advanced knowledge of therapies for chronic and disabling conditions of adults and children.
Program planning. The process by which administrators assess needs and develop plans to meet those needs.

REFERENCES

1. American Dietetic Association. "Position of the American Dietetic Association: The Roles of Registered Dietitians and Dietetic Technicians, Registered, in Health Promotion and Disease Prevention." *J Am Diet Assoc* 106 (2006): 1875–1884.
2. See Note 1.
3. Kaufman, M. *Nutrition in Promoting the Public's Health: Strategies, Principles, and Practice.* (Sudbury, MA: Jones and Bartlett, 2007).
4. Begley, S. "As America's Waistline Expands, Costs Soar," Reuters news release, April 30, 2012. Accessed January 26, 2013, http://www.reuters.com/article/2012/04/30/us-obesity-idUSBRE83T0C820120430
5. Neelon, S.E.B., and M.E. Briley. "Position of the American Dietetic Association: Benchmarks for Nutrition in Child Care." *J Am Diet Assoc* 111 (2011): 607–615.
6. See Note 5, p. 607.
7. Briggs, M., C.G. Mueller, and S. Fleischhacker. "Position of the American Dietetic Association, School Nutrition Association, and Society for Nutrition Education: Comprehensive School Nutrition Services." *J Am Diet Assoc* 110 (2010): 1738–1749.
8. Academy of Nutrition and Dietetics. Press release, June 14, 2012, media @eatright.org
9. See Note 1.
10. See Note 1.
11. Ward, B. "Compensation and Benefits Survey 2011: Moderate Growth in Registered Dietitian and Dietetic, Registered, Compensation in the Past 2 Years." *J Acad Nutr and Diet* 1 (2012): 29–40.
12. Frank, G.C. *Community Nutrition: Applying Epidemiology to Contemporary Practice.* (Sudbury, MA: Jones and Bartlett, 2008).
13. Public Health Nutrition Practice Group of the American Dietetic Association. *Guidelines for Community Nutrition Supervised Practice Experience.* (Chicago: American Dietetic Association, 2003).
14. American Dietetic Association. *Job Descriptions: Models for the Dietetics Profession.* (Chicago: American Dietetic Association, 2003).

The Consultant in Health Care, Business, and Private Practice

"Entrepreneurs shape the future dietetics practice by pursuing innovative and creative ways of providing nutrition products and services."[1]

OUTLINE

INTRODUCTION

As a result of the 2011 Compensation and Benefits Survey, it was reported that 8 percent of registered dietitians (RDs) and about 3 percent of dietetic technicians, registered (DTRs) indicated their primary practice area was in consultation and business.[2] Many dietitians have found the schedule flexibility and compensation of self-employment attractive alternatives to more traditional positions. An entrepreneurial drive is often the impetus for a professional to become a consultant and/or establish a practice. Others do so because family or other obligations lead to becoming a consultant for a better lifestyle fit.

Healthcare institutions have moved an increasing number of services from inpatient care into outpatient clinics, other community agencies, or home care. Governmental regulations led to the need for nutrition consultants in extended care facilities in the 1970s. Together, these trends have led to the need for a greater number of consultant dietitians rather than full-time employees in an institution.

Three types of consultant practice are discussed in this chapter, and while there are similar characteristics of the successful practitioner as in many of the job requirements, each area is unique in several ways because of the nature of the business or practice. The practice areas are consultants in health care and extended care, such as nursing homes and long-term care institutions; consultants in business; and consultants in private practice.

BECOMING A CONSULTANT

Starting a practice as a consultant requires forethought and planning. Two very helpful publications available to guide the dietitian in planning are Helm's *The Entrepreneurial Dietitian* and *The Competitive Edge*.[3,4]

The first step is self-assessment. Personal characteristics are important because an entrepreneur needs to be self-directed, energetic, and action oriented. Previous working experience in dietetics is very important for the person considering becoming a consultant because a great deal of independent activity and judgment is needed, and success is dependent on having had opportunities to develop these characteristics. A number of questions leading an assessment of a person's readiness for practice are the following[5]:

- Are you a self-starter?
- Are you a risk taker?
- Do you have a positive, friendly interest in others?
- Are you a leader?
- Can you handle responsibility?
- Are you a good organizer?
- Are you able to handle a flexible working schedule?
- Do you make up your mind quickly?
- Can people rely on you?
- Can you handle reversals and downturns in business?

A professional making a career change to consulting may need to update his or her resume. It is important to tailor the resume in a way that emphasizes experience and professional qualifications, highlighting those skills that pertain most closely to the position being planned. The resume should be concise; should use strong action verbs; and should be specific about past experiences. Examples of resumes for several different career areas are shown by Matthieu.[6]

The interview will be a next important step after the resume has been sent and after one or more call-backs from interested clients. A professional attitude and appearance make a good first impression. Some advance research about the company or facility will help to formulate additional questions and show interest. Discussion of the amount of time, contracts, and pay should come in the later part of the interview.[7]

Networking with other successful dietitians through one or more practice groups is an excellent way of gaining valuable start-up information. Mentors may be found and networks established from these contacts. Professional liability insurance should be considered early in the planning stage. This insurance is available through the office of the Academy of Nutrition and Dietetics. Networking is also a way of obtaining accounts or positions. Initiating contacts with a healthcare facility or business is followed by a meeting with the administrator and other key personnel. Negotiations should include a clear understanding of the amount of time the consultant will be needed. Although regulations in a healthcare institution may require a dietetic consultant only a small number of hours per month, there may be compelling reasons for more time to be spent in the facility. For instance, in institutions with a large number of residents or in institutions in which a number of residents require skilled care, additional consultation time may well be needed.

Contracts and Fees

Major considerations for the dietitian in consultation and private practice are setting prices and fees and obtaining reimbursement for services. These will be spelled out in the contract, which is a legal document outlining the obligations between the parties involved.[8] Establishing and negotiating the ground rules are important in the initial stages of the process.

Consultants can gain information about reimbursement rates by researching pay levels in the area and region for different types of consulting work and for basic salary levels. Networking with others in a practice group is a good way of obtaining information regarding typical fees. Dietitians who receive reimbursement from insurers or hospitals for medical nutrition therapy will be guided by medical nutrition therapy (MNT) codes establishing payment for treatments authorized by Medicare.[9]

Expenses such as liability insurance, mileage, travel, and any educational components needed should be added to the base pay to arrive at a fee.[10] A helpful discussion on the process of setting fees is presented in *The Entrepreneurial Nutritionist.*[11]

THE CONSULTANT IN HEALTH CARE AND EXTENDED CARE

The role of the consultant in healthcare facilities and extended care became important with the enactment of the Medicare regulations by the Health Care Financing Administration (now called the Centers for Medicare and Medicaid Services or CMS). The Omnibus Reconciliation Act of 1987, amended in 1990 and 1993, provided regulations for nutritional care in long-term facilities that received federal Medicare funds.[12] These facilities (primarily nursing homes) were required to hire a qualified dietitian; as a result, the demand for consultant dietitians rapidly increased from a limited employment area with a short history, few guidelines, and dietitians on their own insofar as job requirements and benefits were concerned. Consultation in healthcare facilities became areas in which many dietitians soon found employment. The opportunities helped many dietitians who had been out of the workforce to return to practice. Some of these dietitians needed to be updated in practice knowledge and skills and turned to continuing education opportunities to refresh themselves on necessary information to practice. Today, many dietitians work as consultants in nursing homes and small hospitals funded by federal and state agencies.

Federal regulations state that the consultant's visits should be of "sufficient frequency to meet the food and nutrition needs of residents in the facility."[13] In many facilities, this meant a minimum of 8 hours a month. While the federal regulations were vague in regard to the actual amount of time required, many states, through licensing, require a minimum of 8 hours. A dietitian contracts with a facility for the amount of time needed, at or above the minimum, to meet the facility's needs.

Some consultants contract with more than one facility and may thereby work part-time or full-time as they choose. Some dietitians are employed full-time for a multifacility chain or in one large facility.

Regulations

A consultant must be familiar with state and federal regulations that apply to long-term or extended care facilities. The health department in each state can provide copies of both regulations. Federal regulations are precise concerning both the physical plant the operation and staffing of the facility. Each facility has its own procedures and set of regulations governing operations. The consultant needs to be thoroughly familiar with these as well as the policies and goals of the facility.

All healthcare providers in the United States need to be familiar with the Health Insurance Portability and Accountability Act (HIPAA) of 1996, as this set of rules concerning rights of patients and clients must be addressed and clients notified of the facility's privacy procedures.[14]

Areas of Practice

Long-term facilities include nursing homes, skilled nursing facilities, subacute care centers, adult day care, residential care facilities, and alcohol and drug rehabilitation facilities. Long-term care facilities may be owned privately, by the cities or counties, by religious organizations, or by corporations. They may be for profit or not for profit; the number of beds varies.

Consultants also may be hired to visit developmentally disabled clients in their homes. In addition, some state health departments contract with consultants to provide services for Women, Infants, and Children (WIC) participants. Other consultants work in home health care, congregate feeding sites, senior citizen centers, correctional facilities, group homes for the developmentally disabled, hospice programs, and small rural hospitals. Adult day care, group homes, and retirement communities are other facilities offering opportunities for the consultant dietitian in health care.

Roles and Responsibilities

A consultant functions in an advisory capacity within a facility; however, he or she has ethical and professional responsibilities for the nutritional care of the residents. Ethical practice issues must be guided by the academy's code of ethics. Professional responsibilities are delineated in the *ADA Standards of Practice for Professional Performance for Registered Dietitians in Nutrition Care*[15] and the *ADA Standards of Practice of Practice and Standards of Professional Performance for Registered Dietitians (Competent, Proficient, and Expert) in Extended Care Settings*.[16] By developing rapport and using organizational skills, the consultant is able to accomplish the needed tasks. Because he or she is usually not in the facility full-time, the day-to-day supervision of dietary services may be provided by a DTR or a dietetic manager.

When a consultant begins employment in a facility, one of the first activities should be a needs assessment of the food and nutrition services for the residents. This assessment will guide further planning and action. Documentation of observations and plans for future visits are very important, beginning with the first visit. The typical activities a consultant performs during a visit to a facility include the following:

- Conferring with the dietary manager and the administrator about day-to-day operations and any problems that need to be addressed during the visit

- Performing nutrition assessment of new residents and conducting a follow-up for all others
- Checking at-risk residents and making recommendations for further nutritional care as indicated. This includes noting unexplained changes in weight or the development of pressure ulcers, checking those on tube feedings, and noting signs of dehydration or otherwise poor nutritional status
- Observing the meal service and eating a meal to evaluate food quality
- Making nutrition rounds and visiting the group dining area at meal time to observe the residents' acceptance of the food and their food intake
- Conducting educational in-service sessions for employees and exchange information regarding departmental activities
- Documenting all activities with any recommendations for follow-up

The consultant may be responsible for developing policy and procedure manuals for the quality improvement program, for safety and sanitation procedures, and for budget management. The reference diet manual should be reviewed and signed by the chief of the medical staff at least annually and should be updated regularly. Consultants may also teach dietetic technician students, conduct classes for the dietary manager, and serve as a preceptor for students in supervised experiences in long-term care.

Standards for Quality Assurance

The Dietetics in Health Care Communities dietetic practice group developed standards of practice in 2011 as a guide for quality assurance in practice.[17] The standards specify areas of activity with examples of outcomes. They include the provision of services, application of research, communication and application of knowledge, utilization and management of resources, and continued competence and professional accountability.

Through written documentation, consultant dietitians can verify actual performance and implement action to meet the expected outcomes. The standards also help develop a workable plan to help consultants meet the responsibilities for which they have been contracted and to evaluate their own knowledge, clinical experience, and management expertise.

THE CONSULTANT IN BUSINESS PRACTICE

An increasingly popular area of practice for the dietitian with an entrepreneurial drive is in business and nontraditional career areas. Potential practice areas identified by the Nutrition Entrepreneurs practice group include services for individuals, corporations, the media, restaurants, food companies, Internet and business technology, sports and health facilities, and coaching. Other areas are in pharmaceutical sales, medical and institutional equipment sales, catering, chefs' schools, and specialized clinics.

Dietitians who work as consultants in businesses of all kinds like to take on new challenges and are often described as risk-takers in new areas of practice. They are energetic and versatile individuals with backgrounds and experience preparing them for innovative roles—roles they may even be required to create. Although many of the responsibilities of a consultant may be similar to those for a full-time dietitian, one of the main differences is often the duration of the assignment. In an established business, the consultant may be given a short-term contract with an identified scope of work and specific deliverables (outcomes). The scope of services is usually an assignment to set up or improve the business practices of the client. It also may be a specific project with a defined beginning and end time period. Examples of activities the consultant may perform include evaluating staffing patterns, establishing an inventory and cost-control system, planning a new production or service system, recommending equipment purchases, and establishing a computerized control system.

Areas of Practice

Business consulting firms at times employ entry-level dietitians for consulting, but usually in a defined scope of responsibility. More often, the dietitian is experienced in some area (e.g., as a clinical dietitian in a healthcare facility or manager of a food service system). The dietitian also may have worked as an assistant to another dietitian for a food processor equipment manufacturer, publisher, marketing company, or software company. When hired, he or she may first be assigned to a team leader to work on a specific part of a major project. With experience, there may be opportunities to expand into other nontraditional roles such as facility management, accounting, design, sales, or marketing. The range of expended responsibility is dependent on the scope of the services performed by the company and those that the dietitians can develop for the company.

The following guidelines can be used by those who may be thinking of moving into management with the goal of consultation in business, private practice, or health care:

- Consider one's personal qualifications to act independently
- Seek advice from a veteran manager or other mentors
- Join a practice group for networking and sharing
- Become familiar with the mission and goals of the business or health-care organization
- Keep up-to-date with the professional literature and continuing education opportunities
- Take advantage of the evidence-based library resources
- Consider further education if advancement and pay would benefit
- Attend professional seminars and meetings
- Be familiar with and apply all aspects of ethical practice
- Match job requirements with education and experience
- Be proficient in the use of technology
- Seek ways to constantly evaluate personal performance

The Dietitian in Private Practice

Many dietitians today become entrepreneurs and enter private practice for a variety of reasons. Some seek new and innovative opportunities out of choice; others do so due to circumstances that make private practice an attractive choice. Examples of the latter might be the loss of a job or the need to work varying hours because of family responsibilities. Opportunities for women in the business world are unquestionably increasing. The healthcare industry continues to downsize from large, centralized centers to outpatient and community centers with fewer staff. Many dietitians seek greater independence and new challenges and, along with a business climate that encourages entrepreneurs, find satisfying careers in private practice.

Not all consultants start a business. Some work at home and combine home and family responsibilities with part-time, contract-type work such as writing, preparing marketing and educational materials, computer searches, and home visits. If a decision is made to open an office, appropriate equipment must be obtained, and secretarial help, as well as other assistants or an office manager, will need to be considered.

Starting a Practice

Cross[18] provides a helpful checklist for starting up in private practice. The first step, she points out, is to maintain an updated file of one's professional credentials and achievements. Regarding references, both giving and receiving employment references may present important issues to be considered.[19] Obtaining state licensure or certification and keeping professional credentials up to date helps establish qualifications. Secondly, joining the state association, dietetic practice groups, and specialty groups, if applicable, will provide opportunities for networking. Becoming involved in local business groups or taking business classes helps one learn the business climate.

Creating a vision and finding one's focus, then creating the road map or business plan, is the next step.[20] The business plan should incorporate the mission and vision statement, product or service to be provided, a description of the target market, the competition, and financial projections. Identifying where to find professional support from an accountant, a banker, a marketing specialist, an information technology specialist, and perhaps a lawyer will provide valuable assistance. Banks, investment companies and community small-business start-up programs often provide advice to assist entrepreneurs in starting a business.

Establishing the business basics by estimating expenses, obtaining necessary insurance, and writing policies and procedures are important steps. A marketing program and a quality-assurance program will help launch and maintain the business. The benefits that can be realized from careful planning include seeing clients succeed and realizing a business profit.

The dietitian who enters private practice needs to possess confidence, determination, perseverance, and the motivation to remain current on trends and changes in the profession and the business world. Remaining up to date comes in great part through taking advantage of continuing education opportunities. The Nutrition Entrepreneurs practice group advises anyone going into private practice—whether to write a book, start a business, become a speaker or coach, or use the Internet to market or provide products and services—to find help through a mentor, and it offers participation in a mentorship program.

Areas of Practice

The consultant in private practice usually will be located outside an organization, but also may be an intrapreneur, or one within an organization who develops new ideas or services that are used profitably in some way. The potential work settings are as diverse as the practitioner's interests and expertise as well as the market demand. This variety is illustrated in **Table 9-1**.

Table 9-1. Settings for Consulting in Private Practice

Private office
Media and communications
Private home
Grocery stores
Physician's or other allied health professional's offices
Restaurants and culinary industry
Corporate settings of work sites
Home health care
Business and industry
Health/fitness/wellness centers and spas
Food companies
Community-based programs
Hotels and resorts
Schools
Research centers
Hospitals
Medical education consulting firms
Day and group homes
Private specialty clinics (specializing in sports medicine, eating disorders, diabetes, renal diseases, oncology, HIV/AIDS)
Senior citizen centers
Nursing homes
Governmental contracts
Rehabilitation centers
Child development centers
Assisted living facilities
Retirement centers

Source: Adapted from Alexander-Israel, D., and C. Roman-Shriver. In *Dietetics: Practice and Future Trends,* 3rd ed. E.A. Winterfeldt, M.L. Bogle, and L.L. Ebro. (Gaithersburg, MD: Aspen Publishers, 2011), p. 137.

The professional services provided are influenced by the needs of the consumer, the demands and changing environments of health care, changes in regulatory agencies, increased autonomy, and advances in science and technology.[21] As new ideas are disseminated and needs identified, more roles are defined for the private practitioner. Dietitians may form alliances and networks to provide services. By teaming with other professionals, the ability to market services and products and share business expense is enhanced. The opportunities presented through a wider range of contacts also may be increased. Examples of such associations are preferred provider organizations to managed care companies, dietitian networks, and dietitian-independent practice associations. Dietetic practice groups provide a means for networking among professionals.

Practice Roles

Consultants in private practice may teach clients and consumers in areas ranging from wellness and prevention to medical nutrition therapy, business and industry, food service and culinary trades, and writing and media presentation. A list of activities is shown in **Table 9-2** as examples of the types of services that consultants may perform.

Table 9-2. Roles of Consultants in Private Practice

Assessment of nutritional status
Menu evaluation and planning
Recipe evaluation and modification
One-on-one counseling
Family counseling
Group counseling
Monitoring of nutritional intervention
Dietary analysis and evaluation of products
Consultant to agencies, institutions, and programs with nutrition components, such as extended care, school food service, hospitals, government agencies, or clinics
Consultant to professionals (health care, food service, culinary industry)
Consultant to corporations (fitness centers, wellness/health promotion programs, benefits departments)
Writing for the lay public (books, newsletters, magazines, newspaper articles)
Professional publications

(continues)

Table 9-2. Roles of Consultants in Private Practice *(continued)*

Group training, presentations, workshops
Developing nutritious/healthier menu items for restaurants
Restaurant and culinary staff training
Assistance in marketing nutrition in restaurants
Computer/software programming (quality management, nutrition education, food service, clinical nutrition)
Developing and marketing nutrition education programs (private and public)
Supermarket tours and grocery information guides
Nutrition labeling information
Rehabilitation and sports injury consultation
Nutrition care planning
Monitoring compliance with local, state, federal regulations (long-term care facilities, drug and alcohol centers, prisons)
Developing, administering, and evaluating nutrition standards
Multidisciplinary preventive and therapeutic services
Health coaching

Source: Alexander-Israel, D., and C. Roman-Shriver. In *Dietetics: Practice and Future Trends.* E.A. Winterfeldt, M.L. Bogle, and L.L. Ebro. Aspen Publishers: Gaithersburg, MD; 1998, p. 209.

Practice roles often can be expanded with more training in business, marketing, and communications and with the development of new skills that cross the boundaries into other health professions.[22] For example, dietitians can become proficient at taking blood pressure and body composition measurements in the home care setting; can secure American College of Sports Medicine Exercise Test Technology certification for performing electrocardiogram-monitored stress tests in sports medicine clinics, or Clinical Laboratory Certification for blood analysis; or can use phlebotomy skills in wellness programs.

Continually emerging roles demand expansion of the dietitian's scope of practice and skills and capitalizing on the talents that are unique to dietitians. Among these are the ability to apply food and nutrition knowledge, use nutrition assessment tools, apply lifestyle-change education to prevent or manage disease, and to collect data on outcomes of nutrition intervention on quality of life and overall care costs.

ETHICAL AND LEGAL BASES OF PRACTICE

The *Code of Ethics for the Profession of Dietetics* is the primary document governing ethical practice in all areas of dietetics. This document, along with any applicable rules or statutes of practice, including licensure from state and local authorities, should be familiar to all consultants. These guidelines will clarify the responsibilities to the public, to clients, to the profession, and to colleagues and other professionals. Feeney[23] offers practical tips for the dietitian applying the code to ethical practice when questions or conflicts arise. Grandgenett[24] gives specific case examples of ethical dilemmas in business practice with discussion of ways they can be handled.

As discussed earlier, the consultant may need to retain legal advice at the outset in order to negotiate a contract and other job-related provisions. The contract is a legal document that guides the consultants scope of practice and may serve as a template for later functions. All consultants should carry personal liability insurance to protect against the possibility of legal action arising out of job-related activities.

SUMMARY

Traditional institutional roles for dietitians, especially in clinical dietetics, are still predominant practice settings; however, many dietitians are using their clinical background to become entrepreneurs in their own practice. The dietitian who possesses the needed personal attributes and the initiative and creativity needed for entrepreneurial success may find a rewarding new career in consultation in healthcare facilities, businesses, or private practice.

DEFINITIONS

Client. The recipient of services or products.

Consultant. A skilled and knowledgeable person qualified to give expert professional advice.

Entrepreneur. An innovative person who initiates a new activity, career, or business.

Intrapraneur. A person within an organization who develops new ideas or services.

Long-term care. Assistance provided over time to people with chronic health conditions and/or physical disabilities and those who are unable to care for themselves.

Managed care. A system of care administered by an entity outside a hospital or healthcare institution in which access, cost, and quality of care are controlled by direct intervention before or during service for purposes of creating efficiencies and/or reducing costs.

Nutrition assessment. Evaluation of an individual's nutritional status based on anthropometric, biochemical, clinical, and dietary information.

Private practice. Self-employment in which a person manages his or her own working career.

Quality improvement. The provision of service that assures the needs of those served are met through adherence to high standards of care.

REFERENCES

1. Academy of Nutrition and Dietetics. *Nutrition Entrepreneurs Dietetic Practice Group.* (2012).
2. Ward, B. "Compensation and Benefits Survey 2011: Moderate Growth in Registered Dietitian and Dietetic Technician, Registered, Compensation in the Past 2 Years." *J Acad Nutr and Diet* 112 (2012): 29–40.
3. Helm, K.K. *The Entrepreneurial Nutritionist,* 4th ed. (Lake Dallas, TX: K.K. Helm Publications, 2010).
4. Helm, K.K. *The Competitive Edge. Advanced Marketing for Dietetic Professionals,* 3rd ed. (Chicago: The Academy of Nutrition and Dietetics: 2009).
5. Adapted from Cross, A.T. "Practical and Legal Considerations of Private Nutrition Practice." *J Am Diet Assoc* 95 (1995): 21–29.
6. Matthieu, J. "Revamping Your Resume for Your Specialty." *J Am Diet Assoc* 110 (2010): 353–355.
7. McCafree, J. "Contract Basics: What a Dietitian Should Know." *J Am Diet Assoc* 103 (2003): 429–440.
8. Peregrin, T. "From Contracts to Clean Claim: Guidelines for Getting Paid." *J Am Diet Assoc* 110 (2010): 837–839.
9. Bender, T. "2009 Medicare MNT Payment Information." *Ventures* XXV, no. 4 (2009): 10.
10. Marcasan, W. "Setting Fees—Where Do I Start?" *J Am Diet Assoc* 111 (2011): 192.
11. See Note 3.

12. Omnibus Budget Reconciliation Act 1987. Amended 1990, 1993.

13. "Skilled Nursing Facilities: Standards for Certification and Participation in Medicare and Medicaid Programs." Federal Register 39 (1974): 22–38.

14. U.S. Department of Health and Human Services. "The Health Insurance Portability and Accountability Act of 1996 (HIPAA) Privacy and Security Rules," Accessed May 1, 2012, www.hhs.gov

15. American Dietetic Association Quality Management Committee. "American Dietetic Association Revised 2008 Standards of Practice for Registered Dietitians in Nutrition; Standards of Professional Practice for Registered Dietitians; Standards of Practice for Dietetic Technicians, Registered, in Nutrition Care; and Standards of Professional Performance for Dietetic Technicians, Registered." *J Am Diet Assoc* 108 (2008): 1538–1542.

16. Roberts, L., S.C. Cryst, G.E. Robinson, C.H. Robinson, C.H. Elliott, L.C. Moore M. Rybicki, and M.P. Carlson. "American Dietetic Association: Standards of Practice and Standards of Professional Performance for Registered Dietitians (Competent, Proficient, and Expert) in Extended Care Settings." *J Am Diet Assoc* 111 (2011): e617–624, e627.

17. See Note 16.

18. Cross, M. "Getting Started in Private Practice: A Checklist to Your Entrepreneurial Path." *J Am Diet Assoc* 108 (2008): 21–24.

19. Zackin, F.M. "Employment References—Giving and Receiving." *J Am Diet Assoc* 1089 (2008): 1053–1055.

20. See Note 8.

21. ADA. "The Role of Dietetics Professionals in Health Promotion and Disease Prevention." *J Am Diet Assoc* 102 (2002): 1680–1687.

22. See Note 6.

23. Feeney, M.J. "When Ethics Collide: An independent Dietetic Consultant's Perspective on Balancing Professional Ethics with the Wishes of Your Client." *J Am Diet Assoc* 108 (2008): 29–31.

24. Grandgenett, R. "Ethics in Business Practice." *J Am Diet Assoc* 110 (2010): 1103–1104.

CHAPTER 10

Career Choices in Business and Health and Wellness

"The ancient Greeks attained a high level of civilization based on good nutrition, regular physical activity, and intellectual development."[1]

OUTLINE

- Introduction
- The Dietitian in Business and Communications
  - Career Opportunities
  - Mentors and Networks
  - Strategic Skill Building
- The Dietitian in Health and Wellness Programs
  - Sports Nutrition
  - Cardiovascular Nutrition
  - Wellness and Health Promotion
  - Disordered Eating
- Practice Groups
- Summary
- Definitions
- References

INTRODUCTION

Hospitals and extended care facilities are the work settings for the largest percentage of dietitians and dietetic technicians; however, there are many career choices available in other settings. Consultation and private practice were discussed in a previous chapter. In this chapter, three other areas of dietetic practice opportunity are presented: business, communications, and health and wellness programs.

THE DIETITIAN IN BUSINESS AND COMMUNICATIONS

Following a career path in business and communications has generally been considered a nontraditional choice for dietitians. The American Dietetic Association membership survey in 2011 showed that about 31 percent of dietitians work in the for-profit sector, including those in contract food management, managed care organizations, and other for-profit organizations.[2] The for-profit category also represents a wide range of positions, including private practice, owning a business, and working with corporations, trade associations, food and pharmaceutical companies, and hotels and restaurants.

Expanded opportunities in business and communications are expected to continue and grow as employers add dietitians to their organization by realizing their value to the business. The major reasons appear to be to increase the company's credibility, to promote customer health and nutrition, and to increase the understanding of customer needs. Given the current trends reported by the Food Marketing Institute, consumers believe the main payoffs of good health are being more active, relieving stress, lowering disease risk, having more energy, and living longer.[3] Food producers, food retailers, and food service establishments take note of what is important to the public and respond by providing products that help meet nutritional needs. Food labeling laws, healthy vending programs, the 2012 farm bill, food safety regulations, and other governmental initiatives are helping to position good nutrition within closer reach of people.

Career Opportunities

There are many paths to a career in business and communications for interested and qualified dietitians (**Table 10-1**). The importance of early exposure to the business world is increasingly recognized, as pointed

Table 10-1. Career Opportunities in Business and Communications

Food Industry
  Food and beverage manufacturing and distributing
  Market research companies
  Trade associations
  Hotels and restaurants
  Contract food service companies
  Commodity groups such as the pork, beef, and egg producers
  National associations
    National Dairy Association
    National Livestock and Meat Board
    Food Marketing Institute
    Grocery Manufacturers
Communications
  Freelance writing
  Writing for publications or newsletters
  Public relations and advertising
  Media spokesperson
  Computer training
  Internet education and services
Health Industry Groups
  Worksite wellness programs
  Health clubs and spas
  Pharmaceutical companies
  Nutritional product and dietary supplement companies
  Heart, cancer, and diabetes associations

out in recommendations that dietetics students experience a rotation in a business environment as part of their undergraduate study, dietetic internship, or graduate study.[4] Students and supervisors can discover opportunities by contacting exhibitors at professional meetings, local businesses, or by contacting other professionals in business and communications. A business rotation may also offer the opportunity for exposure to marketing and public relations activities that are essential in business.

The Dietitians in Business and Communications practice group identifies its members as presidents, vice presidents, food service directors, food stylists, researchers, consultants, sales managers, marketing managers, restaurateurs, test kitchen managers, and software specialists.

How does an individual get a start in business? Several steps are important, including the following[5]:

- Make a list of your talents and interests.
- Make a list of all the possible areas into which you could work, including, but not limited to, writing, speaking, publishing, research, marketing, teaching, sales, media, cooking demonstrations, counseling, coaching, managing, catering, and product development.
- Make a list of the groups with whom you enjoy working and/or in which you have had some experience.
- Read newsletters and journals—the *Academy of Nutrition and Dietetics Journal*, dietetic practice group newsletters, and other publications—and make a list of dietitians doing things you would enjoy doing.
- Contact those working in the areas of interest.
- Network, network, network!

Dietitians in business and communications cite several positive things they like about their jobs, including challenging work, learning opportunities, opportunity for creativity, fast pace, visibility, and remuneration. At the same time, some indicate there can be stress, long hours, a fast pace, bureaucracy, and a lot of information to absorb. The dietitian who is flexible and experienced in the business world is most likely to succeed.

Mentors and Networks

Dietitians traveling a nontraditional path agree that having a mentor, networking, developing a strategic skill set, and keeping current with research and consumer trends are factors necessary to build successful careers. A mentor may be a coworker, an instructor, or another professional. A mentor in the same organization can provide insight into policies, procedures, and the unspoken policies of a company.

Networking both inside and outside the boundaries of dietetics is a way of finding a mentor, gathering information, and connecting with others. The networking offered through dietetic practice groups is invaluable to professionals looking for opportunities for change or advancement in nontraditional areas. Affiliating with other professional associations will provide more ideas and contacts.

Strategic Skill Building

The ability to communicate effectively, along with business know-how and public relations, or people skills, is strategic to a successful career. Industry studies routinely point out that communicating well means the difference between success and failure. The ability to build on earlier education and experience leads to professional growth and enhanced job performance. For example, if a job requires evaluating research and working with research and development, a good grounding in science is important. Clinical education and experience help a dietitian understand the health and nutritional implications when producing and marketing a new food or supplement or educational materials.

Advancing into positions with increasing responsibility and managerial skill may necessitate continuing education, often in the business-related areas of study. The growth of online and distance education helps make this possible even for the professional working full-time or in locations away from the educational setting. Dietitians in business frequently continue their education by acquiring an MBA or an advanced degree in management or finance.

Dietitians in business often establish a website in order to enhance their business image, complement business advertising, attract new clients or customers outside the local area, or to start a new business venture.[6] They may also find this a useful way to learn more about specific businesses and to build networks.

THE DIETITIAN IN HEALTH AND WELLNESS PROGRAMS

Wellness, health promotion, corporate fitness, and sports nutrition programs are all career areas that have developed in recent years. Although both sports and dietetics as professions or areas of interest have existed for centuries, the combination of the two as a career specialty is relatively recent. The growth of wellness and fitness programs has been rapid as the relationship between nutritional status and maintenance of health and prevention of disease becomes more evident.[7]

Diet is a known risk factor for the development of the three chronic diseases that are the leading cause of death in adults in the United States: cancer, cardiovascular disease, and stroke.[8] Additional health problems of adults are also closely associated with diet and eating behaviors, including obesity, diabetes, high blood pressure, and osteoporosis. The numbers of deaths and medical costs can be significantly altered by changes in diet and lifestyle when it is considered that billions of dollars are spent each year on schemes and unproven methods to reduce body weight and prevent cancer, not to mention the money spent treating adults with these diseases and their complications.

Reports from the National Health and Nutrition Examination Survey III (NHANES) indicate an alarming increase in the prevalence and severity of obesity in young children, older children, and adolescents, as well as adults.[9] These statistics point to the need for programs in health promotion, wellness, fitness, and the prevention and treatment of obesity, which greatly expands career options for dietitians.

Some dietitians have developed their own programs through practice and research and now market or license the programs to other dietitians and health professionals, both nationally and internationally. Others continue to work in hospitals, ambulatory care centers, clinics, rehabilitation centers, and athletic clubs or gyms. Those in private practice provide counseling and medical nutrition therapies aimed at preventing and treating obesity.

Even with, or perhaps because of, the increasing prevalence of obesity, many dietary fads, drugs, and questionable dieting programs have escalated and consume enormous amounts of money each year. This phenomenon emphasizes the need and opportunities that exist for dietitians and other health professionals in this area.

Sports Nutrition

Interest in sports and cardiovascular nutrition among members of the ADA led to the formation of the Sports, Cardiovascular and Wellness Nutrition dietetic practice group. Disordered eating as an area of practice was added to the group to include dietary professionals with an interest in disordered eating (such as anorexia nervosa and bulimia), as they recognized the frequent presence of eating disorders among athletes and the critical role that the identification and treatment of disordered eating has in maintaining health and wellness.

The American Dietetic Association, the Dietitians of Canada, and the American College of Sports Nutrition issued a position paper in 2009 concerning nutrition and athletic performance.[10] The importance of optimal nutrition and the roles and responsibilities of healthcare professionals were discussed in the paper. The educational needs of those aspiring to be sports nutritionists were detailed in an article by Clark.[11] Knowledge of nutrition and exercise science knowledge, business skills, and a foundation of strong clinical experience are all important, especially because many sports nutritionists are entrepreneurs. A list of the clinical concerns commonly presented to a sports nutritionist is shown in **Table 10-2**.

Dietetic professionals with a specialty in sports nutrition can be found in a wide variety of settings, from sports medicine clinics to professional football/basketball teams, from high school athletics to the Olympics, and from universities to fitness centers. Many incorporate sports nutrition into their more general practice of nutrition counseling or private practice. Today, several professional sports teams include dietitians as paid consultants

Table 10-2. Clinical Concerns Commonly Presented to a Sports Nutritionist

Allergies	Diarrhea
Alcohol addiction	Gastric reflux
Amenorrhea	Gout
Anemia	Headaches
Anorexia	Hypoglycemia
Arteriosclerosis	Hyperlipdemia
Binge eating	Hypertension
Body image distortion	Menopause
Bulimia	Obesity/overweight
Cancer (prevention, recovery from)	Osteoporosis
Chronic fatigue	Pregnancy/perinatal nutrition
Constipation	Stress fractures
Diabetes	Surgery (special nutritional needs pre- and postoperative)

Source: Reprinted from Journal of the American Dietetic Association 100, Number 12 (December 2000), Clark, N. "Identifying the Educational Needs of Aspiring Sports Nutritionists," 1522–1524, Copyright 2000, with permission from Elsevier.

whose expertise serves to enhance the players' performance. A few professional athletes have employed personal dietitians primarily to help them maintain appropriate body weight and ratio of fat to lean body mass.

Some dietitians specialize as nutrition trainers for college athletes and teams in the sport or sports in which they have the greatest personal interest, such as swimming, wrestling, baseball, or cycling.

Many dietetic professionals working in the area of sports nutrition also work as clinical dietitians for acute care facilities, as outpatient dietitians, or in private practice in nutrition consulting. In addition, some dietitians are employed to supervise the food production and training tables in college athletic residence halls. Some professional athletes seek information on diet during the off-season to maintain body weight and strength. As part of his or her daily routine, a sports nutritionist may counsel athletes one on one regarding their food intake and appropriate nutrients or their use of dietary supplemental aids.[12] A nutritionist may also conduct group classes on low-fat eating at a fitness center or work with a high school team to suggest healthful choices for eating when the team travels. Sports nutritionists also serve as part-time staff at health clubs and are available to answer questions members may ask on nutrition or to conduct classes on eating for competition and good health.

An additional career for some dietitians with experience in sports nutrition and fitness has emerged in writing and developing nutrition education materials appropriate for athletes of all ages. Other dietitians enjoy speaking and/or writing for the media and consultative arrangements with any number of organizations. Another career option that is growing emanates from the proliferation of gymnasiums and physical fitness centers for young children and adolescents. Although these gyms and centers were started for tumbling and gymnastic opportunities, there is a need for expertise in nutrition in these settings, especially combined with principles of child development. Parents and consumers are welcoming the dietitian's expertise related to obesity, weight maintenance, and disordered eating patterns in young children and adolescents. In some instances, entrepreneurial dietitians are developing centers and mobile units that go to elementary schools or other sites for demonstrations of appropriate physical activity and the benefits of good food choices and nutrition.

Knowledge of exercise physiology through course work in exercise science is essential if the sports nutritionist combines nutrition and exercise in work with clients. Many dietetic professionals work to enhance their education and expertise by entering graduate programs in exercise physiology, counseling, psychology, or business administration. In addition, although few college or university programs in sports nutrition currently exist, many graduate students choose to conduct research for their thesis or dissertation on a topic directly related to sports nutrition. By acquiring a strong foundation in foods and normal and clinical nutrition with study in a related area, the dietetic student can better prepare him- or herself for practice in sports nutrition.

A thorough list of roles and responsibilities for the sports dietitian is found in the position paper: *Position of the American Dietetic Association, Dietitians of Canada, and the American College of Sports Medicine: Nutrition and Athletic Performance.*[13]

Cardiovascular Nutrition

With the abundance of research continuing in the area of diet and heart disease, as well as the fact that heart disease remains the number one cause of death for Americans, careers in cardiovascular nutrition offer abundant options. Most acute-care facilities whose services include open-heart surgery have cardiac rehabilitation programs in place. These typically include inpatient and outpatient components, both of which offer nutrition counseling and education as part of the program. Cardiac rehabilitation programs offer multidisciplinary teams who deal with all aspects of risk factor reduction, as well as education of the patient and family. Team members may include a medical director, cardiac rehabilitation nurse clinicians, exercise specialist, physical therapist, social worker, occupational therapist, and a dietitian. Education of the patient and family is often conducted in a variety of ways, from individual instruction to group classes. The dietitians may also design and conduct classes on low-fat cooking and other food preparation techniques.

Dietitians who specialize in cardiovascular nutrition may be employed by lipid research clinics. These professionals are responsible for teaching clinic patients how to change their eating habits to lower total fat and saturated fat or to comply with a research feeding protocol. In this setting at a university, they may conduct research on the latest cardiology/nutrition methodologies. Opportunities also exist with pharmaceutical companies as sales representatives or in the public relations departments of large food companies that market products to patients with cardiovascular disease and their families.

Wellness and Health Promotion

The opportunities for dietitians in wellness and health promotion are numerous and diverse. Dietitians who specialize in wellness may have a private practice or consulting business and negotiate contracts with industry, corporations, or health clubs. Others are employed by medical centers or corporations to manage their on-site wellness and health promotion programs, which may include conducting classes for employees, developing incentives to foster a greater interest in exercise and nutrition, and increasing productivity by helping to reduce employee illness. Because nutrition is part of wellness, dietitians specializing in wellness and health promotion also may be involved in programs on smoking cessation, meditation and yoga, stress management, exercise, back safety, and employee relations.

Corporations and large institutions initially began providing work-site wellness programs for their employees because research and reports showed that these programs improved employee health, increased productivity, and decreased absenteeism and lost work days due to illness. As these programs developed and increased in numbers across the country in businesses of all sizes, data began to accumulate on the economic benefits of work-site wellness programs. With healthcare costs soaring and major changes occurring in healthcare and insurance coverage, employers were eager to explore wellness and health promotion programs that would save the corporation money. The common method for defining economic benefits is through the benefit–cost ratio in which the cost is the actual dollar cost of providing the program, and benefits are expressed in dollars saved from reduced absenteeism, disability expenses, and medical costs.

The ability to work as a facilitator and to conduct classes in a group setting is an important characteristic of the successful wellness professional. Counseling skills are also necessary because dealing with high-risk persons may be a regular aspect of the job. In addition, the dietitian must be prepared to analyze and evaluate enormous amounts of information available to employees and clients through media routes. This counseling may take place in groups, individually, at health fairs, over the telephone, or via computers.

Wellness and fitness programs are also emerging for increasing numbers in the aging and retied population as well as the younger employed groups. Research indicates that even though aging is inevitable, biologic aging can be delayed through appropriate nutrition and exercise.[14] As the number of senior citizens increases, this will provide another career opportunity for dietitians specializing in health promotion. Fitness programs to improve the quality of life and encourage wellness in this age group including nutrition, exercise, and lifestyle changes are developing.

Several national organizations provide excellent and accurate information for dietitians seeking up-to-date knowledge on wellness and health promotion programs and concepts. In addition, all have information on the Internet. The major organizations with this information are the following:

- The Academy of Nutrition and Dietetics (www.eatright.org)
- International Food Information Council (http://www.ific.us/)
- National Institutes of Health (www.nih.gov)
- Centers for Disease Control and Prevention (www.cdc.gov)
- American College of Sports Medicine (www.ascm.org)
- American Alliance on Health, Physical Education, Recreation, and Dance (www.aahperd.org)
- Food and Nutrition Information Center (http://fnic.nal.usda.gov)

The Internet also offers the opportunity and challenge for the individual dietitian to develop websites and disseminate nutrition and fitness messages by this means.

Disordered Eating

Dietitians who specialize in disordered eating work in a variety of settings, including residential treatment centers, hospitals (both medical and psychiatric), outpatient clinics, managed care organizations, university health centers, and private practice. The specialty of disordered or problematic eating encompasses several areas in which nutritional, physical, and psychological issues are intertwined with eating behavior, such as obesity, chronic dieting, anorexia nervosa, bulimia nervosa, compulsive eating, and binge eating disorders. Complications of these disorders are potentially life threatening. Many have their origin or manifestation in childhood or adolescence. Although most of these disorders affect adolescent females, there have been some reports of similar behavior in males. Effective treatment of disordered eating requires knowledge and skills in counseling, cognitive behavioral therapy, family systems theory, addiction, and pharmacology.[15]

Because of the biopsychosocial nature of disordered eating, the role of the dietitian on the treatment team is vital. The dietitian educates the client about food, physical activity, and body size and shape and guides him or her in developing a sound eating style and physical activity pattern. Clients may share their thoughts and feelings about food, weight, and physical activity with the dietitian. They may also share life situations and events that are stressful for them, such as a job change, marital problems, school problems, relationships, and burnout. The dietitian helps clients identify how stress affects their eating style and how they feel about food, their body size and shape, and physical activity. Ongoing communication with the treatment team therapist, psychiatrist, and physician is essential so that the dietitian can discern which issues are nutrition related and which are psychological or medical. It takes years of experience for the dietitian to most effectively complement his or her skills and expertise with other members of the team.

Dietitians working in programs to treat disordered eating benefit from regular supervision from a mental health professional who specializes in problematic eating. This relationship provides a forum for discussion of specific cases, as well as helps to clarify which issues are appropriately addressed in nutrition therapy versus psychotherapy. Furthermore, many dietitians seek continuing education in areas such as women's issues, cognitive behavioral therapy, family counseling, psychotherapeutic counseling skills, and psychopharmacology. The intention is to sharpen counseling skills and enhance the understanding of sociological and psychological aspects of disordered eating while consistently staying within the scope of practice of the dietetic professional, adhering to the standards of practice and professional performance and the academy's code of ethics.[16,17]

PRACTICE GROUPS

Dietitians in business typically join the Dietitians in Business and Communications practice group, the Management in Food and Nutrition Systems practice group, the Food and Culinary Professionals practice group, and the Nutrition Entrepreneurs practice group. By joining one or more of the groups, members are able to benefit from networking, mentoring, information exchange, professional enhancement, and leadership opportunities.

Most practice groups offer their members continuing education programs, periodic newsletters, forums for exploring practice issues, and innovative products and services. In addition, the appropriate standards of practice and standards of professional performance provide guidance and information about what is expected of dietetic professionals in these areas of practice.[18,19]

Dietitians in health and wellness programs have a number of choices among the various clinical groups, with the Sports, Cardiovascular, and Wellness Nutrition group likely the primary choice. Others are Behavioral Health Nutrition and Weight Management. Standards of practice and professional performance are available for these areas as well.[20,21]

SUMMARY

The dietitian in business and communications often deals with the public in visible and varied ways. The opportunities in these areas continually expand as consumers become increasingly aware of the health benefits of good food choices and seek valid information.

Dietitians with expertise in worksite wellness, sports and cardiovascular nutrition, and disordered eating are increasingly in demand in nontraditional settings. They must be creative and adept in the promotion of healthy eating behaviors. In addition, nutrition education must be presented in a manner that is directly usable by consumers. The dietitians may also be able to translate scientific information into user-friendly terms.

DEFINITIONS

Anorexia nervosa. An eating disorder in which preoccupation with dieting and thinness leads to excessive weight loss.

Bulimia nervosa. An eating disorder involving frequent episodes of binge eating and nearly always followed by purging, again leading to weight loss.

Cardiovascular nutrition. Application of medical nutrition therapy for those with heart and blood vessel conditions or to prevent the diseases.

Disordered eating. Abnormal eating patterns.

Health promotion. Education and preventive measures directed toward basically healthy populations to foster wellness.

Networking. Activities directed toward making connections with others through varied contacts.

Sports nutrition. The area of nutrition specific to the needs of those who participate in sports activities.

Wellness. State of optimal health and the absence of disease.

REFERENCES

1. Simopoulos, A. "A Declaration of Olympia on Nutrition and Fitness." *Nutr Today* 3 (1996): 250–252.
2. Ward, B. "Compensation and Benefits Survey 2011: Moderate Growth in Registered Dietitian and Dietetic Technician, Registered, Compensation in the Past 2 Years." *Acad Nutr and Diet J* 112 (2012): 29–40.
3. Food Marketing Institute. "Trends in the United States: Consumer Attitudes and the Supermarket." (2000). Accessed March 19, 2012, www.fmi.org
4. Kapica, C., and J.O.S. Maillet. "A Business Rotation for Dietitians—An Imperative in the New Millennium." *J Am Diet Assoc* 102 (2002): 1220.
5. Indorato, D.A. "Innovative Services by and for Dietitians." *Today's Dietitian* 3 (2001): 16–19.
6. Pangan, T., and C. Bedner. "Dietitian Business Websites: A Survey of Their Profitability and How You Can Make Yours Profitable." *J Am Diet Assoc* 101 (2002): 399–402.
7. Golson, S.K. "Make Time for Daily Physical Activity." *J Am Diet Assoc* 109 (2009): 18.
8. National Center for Health Statistics. "Data 1997–2010." Accessed May 5, 2012, www.cdc.gov
9. Centers for Disease Control and Prevention. "Overweight among Children and Adolescents, 16–19 Years of Age, by Selected Characteristics. U.S. 1963–65 through 2005–2006." Accessed May 5, 2012, www.cdc.gov
10. "Position of the American Dietetic Association, Dietitians of Canada, and the American College of Sports Medicine: Nutrition and Athletic Performance." *J Am Diet Assoc* 109 (2009): 509–527.
11. Clark, N. "Identifying the Educational Needs of Aspiring Sports Nutritionists." *J Am Diet Assoc* 100 (2000): 1522–1524.
12. Shattuck, D. "Sports Nutritionists Feel the Competitive Edge." *J Am Diet Assoc* 101 (2001): 517–518.
13. See Note 10.
14. Etgen, T., D. Sander, U. Huntgeburth, H. Pappas, H. Fasti, and H. Bickel. "Physical Activity and Incident Cognitive Impairment in Elderly Persons." *Arch Intern Med* 170 (2010): 186–193.

15. ADA. "Nutrition Intervention in the Treatment of Eating Disorders," Position paper. *J Am Diet Assoc* 111 (2011): 1236–1241.

16. Tholking, M.M., A.C. Mellowsprings, S.G. Eberle, R.P. Lamb, E.S. Myers, C.S. Scribner, R.F. Sloan, and K.B. Wetherall. "American Dietetic Association: Standards of Practice and Standards of Professional Performance for Registered Dietitians (Competent, Proficient, and Expert) in Disordered Eating and Eating Disorders (DE and ED)." *J Am Diet Assoc* 111 (2011): 1242–1249.

17. American Dietetic Association/Commission on Dietetic Registration. "Code of Ethics for the Profession of Dietetics and Process for Consideration of Ethics Issues." *J Am Diet Assoc* 109 (2009): 1461–1467.

18. See Note 17.

19. American Dietetic Association Quality Management Committee. "American Dietetic Association Revised 2008 Standards of Practice for Registered Dietitians in Nutrition Care: Standards of Professional Performance for Registered Dietitians; Standards of Practice for Dietetic Technicians, Registered, in Nutrition Care; and Standards of Professional Performance for Dietetic Technicians, Registered." *J Am Diet Assoc* 109 (2009): 1538–1542.

20. Steinmuller, P.L., N.L. Meyer, L.K. Fruskall, M.N. Manore, N.R. Rodriguez, M. Macedonio, R.L. Bird, and J.R. Berning. "American Dietetic Association Standards of Practice and Standards of Professional Performance for Registered Dietitians (Generalist, Specialty, Advanced) in Sports Nutrition." *J Am Diet Assoc* 109 (2009): 544–551.

21. Emerson, M.P., P. Kerr, M.D.C. Soler, T.A. Girard, R. Hofflinger, E. Pritchett, and M. Otto. "American Dietetic Association Standards of Practice and Standards of Professional Performance for Registered Dietitians (Generalist, Specialty, and Advanced) in Behavioral Health Care." *J Am Diet Assoc* 106 (2006): 608–613.

CHAPTER 11

The Dietitian as Manager and Leader

"Skills such as team building, delegation, communication, negotiation, and self-management are fundamental to high performance. Fortunately, these can be learned and enhanced through continuing education and training."[1]

OUTLINE

INTRODUCTION

Management is often regarded as the responsibilities and challenges that have to do with being in charge or being the boss of a department, and therefore, the entry-level dietitian often believes that he or she does not need to be concerned with knowing how to manage. In reality, all dietitians, regardless of their job title or job responsibilities, perform many managerial functions and need to develop managerial skills. The clinical dietitian, the food service manager, the nutritionist in community nutrition programs, the educator, the private practitioner, the dietitian in business and industry, and healthcare administrators all perform management functions. Among these functions are setting goals, evaluating outcomes, managing resources, integrating and coordinating personnel activities, training personnel and allied professionals, communicating, and promoting quality control.

Management and leadership have many overlapping characteristics and have been described in several ways by leaders in the management field. A simplified way to view them is to think of management as the activities that go into making a department or an institution run—doing things— and leadership as the qualities a person (a manager) needs to possess in order to make things go right. We could say "things are managed and people are led."[2]

In this chapter, we discuss leadership and management separately, but because many functions are complementary, both need to be developed together. A professional cannot be truly successful unless characteristics of both leadership and management skills are evident in the workplace.

LEADERSHIP

Frank[3] describes leadership as "the art of bringing together people with diverse talents, interests, ideas, and backgrounds to voluntarily participate in a shared approach toward common or compatible goals." This definition makes the distinction between accomplishing tasks and inspiring people to willingly perform those tasks. Leadership consists of the traits that accompany good management skills, and for someone to be successful, the two functions need to go together.

Leaders and thinkers, including Peter Drucker, who is recognized as an authority on leadership, consider that three important characteristics for successful leadership are[4]:

1. Thinking through the mission of the organization, defining it, and establishing it clearly and visibly. The leader sets the goals and priorities and maintains the standards.
2. Viewing leadership as a responsibility and not a rank or a privilege. Effective leaders are rarely permissive, but when things go wrong, they do not blame others. They encourage and help develop strong associates.
3. Earning trust in order to have followers. To trust a leader, it is not necessary to like or to agree; rather trust is the conviction that the leader means what he or she says and has integrity.

Attaining Leadership Skills

A question often debated is whether people are born leaders or whether they develop leadership skills and thereby become leaders. In support of the view that leadership skills can be acquired, several actions that make for leadership development are the following:[5]

- Well-defined values
- Commitment to quality
- Responsive to the consumer, client, and the public
- Stimulating a nurturing work environment
- Creativity and innovation
- Open lines of communication and shared information
- Inclusive process for decision making
- Planning and fostering meaningful change to achieve goals and improved performance

Leadership Development

The American Dietetic Association (ADA) developed the Institute for Leadership in 2003.[6] At a yearly event, members receive training in leadership, dialogue, and sharing perspectives through private, personalized agendas. Interactive breakout sessions and workshops as well as structured networking events have been a part of the annual sessions. A certificate of training is offered at the conclusion of each annual forum.

In reviewing traditional leadership theory, it has been suggested that more information is needed about the way dietitians develop as leaders.[7] Consistent with earlier theories about the way humans grow through stages of mental development and become leaders in predictable ways, a newer theory is that of constructive development, described as an alternative approach to leadership as a way of growing in stages.[8] Studies of leaders across industries and organizational levels show that 5 percent of all leaders are at a stage where they are focused on self and seldom welcome feedback; 80 percent are in a middle stage of avoiding conflict, becoming a member of a group, having a strong belief system and being results and goal oriented; while 15 percent are at the highest stage during which there is systematic problem solving, seeking feedback, realizing the complexity of the environment, and having a deep appreciation of others. When a survey of ADA leaders was conducted in 2006, most were shown to be in the high part of the medium range group. It is suggested that by becoming aware of their own stage, dietitians can develop further in their leadership ability by seeking out a supportive environment, perhaps through advanced study, mentors, supportive coworkers, networking, and others.

Another aspect of leadership is the need for what has become known as emotional intelligence, along with intellectual and technical skills. The most effective leader has a high degree of emotional intelligence. This is defined as self-awareness, self-regulation, motivation, empathy, and social skills. These skills can be learned through experience and internal commitment.[9]

Leadership for Quality and Efficiency

Leadership development programs, increasingly conducted in hospitals and other healthcare organizations, improve both the quality and efficiency of care. Opportunities found to result from three qualitative studies of leadership development are the following[10]:

- Increase the caliber of the workforce
- Enhance efficiency in the organization's education and development activities
- Reduce turnover and related expenses
- Focus organizational attention on specific priorities

Potential activities to improve leadership development are shown in **Table 11-1**.

Table 11-1. Activities to Improve Leadership Development

- Improve the caliber and quality of the workforce by focusing training, providing development in specific areas and creating opportunitoes for application of new skills.

- Enhance efficiency in the organization's education and development activities by providing develpent training and education to reduce travel expense and extend reach of programs.

- Reduce turnover and related expenses through combining leadership activities to employee satisfaction sureys and providing leadership skills to reduce employee dissatisfaction.

- Focus organizational retention on specific priorities through leadership development and education; designing specific educational programs and tying performancve evaluation to organizational goals while making appropriate education and training available to help people meet the goals.

MANAGEMENT FUNCTIONS

Management is usually defined in terms of the traditional functions described by management experts. Although the number of functions vary according to the way in which they are presented, the following six are universally accepted[11]:

1. *Planning.* Planning is the activity of setting goals and objectives. The extent of the planning, from setting broad, long-range goals for a large organization to planning shorter term goals, will usually be determined by where persons are in the organizational hierarchy.
2. *Organizing.* Organizing is the reflection of how the organization accomplishes its goals and objectives. The tasks to be performed, assignment of tasks, allocation of resources, and flow of authority and communication are established.
3. *Coordinating.* Coordinating involves activities that lead to the efficient use of resources to attain the goals and objectives.
4. *Staffing.* Staffing means determining human resource needs, then recruiting, selecting, hiring, and training the necessary staff.
5. *Directing.* Directing (or leading) refers to those activities that enable accomplishment of the organization goals, that communicate those goals, and that create an atmosphere that encourages commitment and desired performance.
6. *Controlling.* Controlling occurs when performance is assessed against standards that have been translated from the goals and objectives and corrective measures applied as needed.

Dietitians who are experienced in management areas of practice are aware that overarching all those activities are the need to communicate effectively—realizing that this is always a two-way process—and to develop the ability to work in productive ways with others in the organization at all levels. Setting goals and standards, incorporating as much technology as feasible and needed, and being financially astute are all critical to successful practice.

SKILLS AND ABILITIES OF MANAGERS

Three fundamental sets of skills needed by managers at various levels to function effectively are human relations skills, technical skills, and conceptual skills (**Figure 11-1**). Earlier traditional views of management held

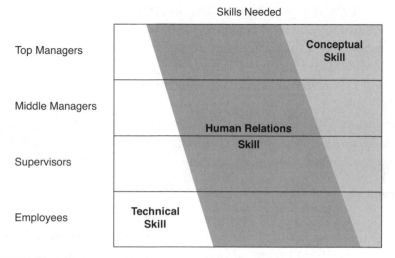

FIGURE 11-1. Balancing Management and Leadership.

Source: R.H. Woods and J.Z. King, Leadership and Management in the Hospitality Industry, Third Ed. (Lansing, Mich: American Hotel & Lodging Educational Institute, 2010, p. 56.

that top managers only primarily needed human relations and conceptual skills, while the more contemporary view is that technical skills as well are increasingly important for the top manager, especially in small organizations and in those with flattened and decentralized organizational patterns. What is immediately apparent from Figure 11-1 is that all levels of managers and even employees need to possess equal amounts of human relations skills that are predominant among the three sets of skills. The need for technical skills increases with lesser overall managerial responsibilities, while the higher conceptual skills decrease. The use of particular skills, such as the need to hire and train new employees or to engage in long-range strategic planning, will vary from day to day with changes in the work environment. The specific activities practiced in these three skill areas are discussed in the following sections.

Human Relations Skills

Interpersonal Relationships

Interpersonal skills are always rated highly when management skills are described or studied. The ability to work with others toward common goals is the number one factor denoting success among healthcare multidepartmental managers.[12] Numerous books and articles have been published about establishing and maintaining interpersonal relationships. Every dietitian will benefit from including one or more in his or her library. The *Harvard Business Review* is also an excellent source for readings in this area.

Generational diversity, or the involvement of several distinct generations in the workplace, presents another aspect of achieving successful working relationships.[13] Different generations of workers are assumed to have different loyalties and expectations resulting in the need for open-mindedness, effective communication, and respect for others on the part of the manager.

Communication

Communication at both individual and group levels will assure that information flow reaches all those in an organization. Keeping others informed, seeking input from others in the organization, and rewarding staff for good work and successes lead to satisfaction and cooperation. Staff members are excellent sources of information, ideas, and solutions and should always be involved when new programs or procedures are being planned. The manager needs to receive information from as many sources as possible and no one in the organization should be overlooked for this input.

In an interesting study among dietitians in Australia, it was pointed out that trust, professionalism, and communications are interrelated.[14] Trust may be defined, in this context, as "confidence in the reliability of persons."[14a] There is better communication between clients and the professional when there is a perception that the dietitian/professional is the expert and can be trusted. A model showing the way these actions work together is shown in Figure 11-1.

The skillful communicator is often one who is also a transformational leader. Such a manager stimulates innovative ways of thinking, can achieve greater performance on the part of those managed, and has vision that can lead to organizational change when needed. By communicating openly and directly with all members of a team, others are motivated to share in commitment to the needs of the group as a whole.[15]

Coaching and Mentoring

Most dietitians will be, at some time in their career, in the position of assisting and supporting a coworker or employee as they learn a new job or develop new skills, and thus will become a coach or mentor. A mentor is described as a person who teaches through verbal instruction, demonstration of particular activities or skills, and role modeling. Coaching is similar in that it is used to inspire and motivate as well as teach. The successful dietitian may function in both these roles in order to accomplish needed tasks. Staff personnel perform at different levels and learn in different ways. It is the enterprising coach or mentor who is able to adapt actions to motivate, encourage, and support staff, thereby creating a productive and harmonious team. Mentoring is discussed in greater detail later in this text.

Managing Conflict

Conflict occurs in any organization and wherever people work in groups. Conflict may arise from competition for resources, overlapping responsibilities, status struggles, poor communications, inadequate training, or differences in values and beliefs. The dietitian who recognizes causes of conflict and assists in taking steps to overcome the differences will be looked to as a manager and leader. When dealt with quickly and constructively, conflict can be a way of improving performance.[16]

Networking

Networking within an organization leads to both communication and cooperation. People form networks for sharing social and business information and to increase professional competence. Sharing information is vital in any organization, and the manager will seek opportunities to network both within and beyond the work unit and will encourage others to also network. Networking with other professionals through the dietetic practice groups of the academy and other groups can lead to personal growth, a greater understanding of practice requirements, and enhanced performance in every area of practice.

Technical Skills

Technical skills are those that require a specialized knowledge of techniques, methods, procedures, and processes that accomplish the work of an organization. Knowing how to access and use technology for communications is a must for all professionals in the modern workplace. Online information is rapidly becoming the means by which professionals remain current. Conferences, workshops, meetings, and classes are offered online, by teleconference, or by similar means using newer technology. Not only is communications technology of increasing importance, but technology related to better and faster job performance benefits both individuals and an organization. To the extent that professionals become experts in the technology needed for their jobs, they will also become mentors and coaches for others.

Technology is used in food production and food service and in all areas of clinical practice. Computerized work schedules, purchasing and inventory control, employee records, and production schedules are examples. These activities point to the need for continual training for all staff and a strong working knowledge of the use of technical equipment of all kinds.

Job Skills

The manager has knowledge of what is required of the workforce to perform in an organization, but does not generally perform the work except on an as-needed basis. However, this knowledge allows the manager to supervise those with the specific skills to fulfill the job requirements. The need to have job know-how is essential to assess performance, meet goals, and ensure quality outputs.

Resource Management

Financial management, including cost controls and budget management, comes to mind first when the management of resources is described as a management function. Resources, however, can also refer to job-related supplies and equipment, staff assistance, and even time and energy. Every dietitian and dietetic technician carries certain responsibilities for managing resources and also may be involved in budgeting and long-range planning for the use of resources.

The importance of including financial management in dietetics programs is emphasized by dietetics program directors. In one survey, educators agreed or strongly agreed with the statement, "Entry-level registered dietitians need to be trained in financial management concepts as well as clinical concepts in order to be competent practitioners."[17]

Benchmarking is a process by which the manager can measure the efficiency of work, the products produced, and the services for comparison and improvement.[18] This process is used in both health care and food services. Performance measures that include financial management, customer service, human resources, and operational activities are evaluated in the benchmarking process. Measurements used provide information that can be compared and used for improvement.

Training and Staff Development

The responsibility for hiring and training personnel is primarily that of upper-level management; however, all professionals will at times help train and develop new employees or other professionals. The team concept often followed in healthcare institutions, food service, and hospitality requires that all members of a team function fully and efficiently. Further, team members must know their job-related roles as well as their expected roles as a team member. Efficiency evolves from knowledge and practice and must be encouraged and assisted by those already experienced within an organization.

Team Building

A team functions in ways that support individual efforts and leads to greater productivity. Teams vary in number, may be formal or informal, and may form in a variety of ways. For instance, a team may be formed within a department or from several departments or disciplines to accomplish more than can be accomplished by individuals. Teams may also be temporary or permanent.

The value of teams lies in sharing knowledge and working toward common goals using the experience and expertise of several people in decision making and problem solving. The manager encourages teams and helps make them effective by arranging for persons to participate and providing for training of team members as needed. Teams function best when they are empowered with authority or legal power to reach a level of self-management.[19]

Work groups of persons working together for a common purpose are often formed. As with teams, they may be formally constituted or may function in an informal way such as a gathering of people to solve daily problems. The group leader has several tasks, which include understanding the internal workings of the group, planning ahead and being proactive, and managing interpersonal relations for group cohesion.

Quality Management

Quality is defined as meeting standards and expectations, sometimes in terms of high quality or above a norm or average. The Quality Management Committee of the academy provides direction for monitoring, developing, approving, evaluating, and maintaining quality management in dietetics. The team members of the group interact with the Scope of Practice Framework committee, the Evidence-Based Practice committee, and the Nutrition Care Process committee. Quality assurance in practice results through the coordinated efforts of these groups.

Dietitians in all areas of practice can monitor their own quality of work through the *Code of Ethics for the Profession of Dietetics*, the standards of professional performance, and the professional development portfolio. The outcome is competent practice and a basis for quality improvement.

In the 2010 Commission on Dietetic Registration practice audit[20], 58 percent of entry-level dietitians indicated they perform quality assurance or performance management.

Every institution, department, business, or professional association strives to produce quality goods, services, and people. Rather than relying on subjective methods to detect quality, most organizations establish performance measures by which they assess and ensure continuous quality. In dietetics, performance standards are in effect and are described in other sections of this book. Food production managers use performance measures to ensure the quality of the food service. Patient satisfaction surveys are used for ongoing assessment of the services received. Clinical outcomes can be measured for quality through specific established indicators. The community nutritionist measures quality by satisfactory outcomes of persons receiving instruction and care. The educator measures outcomes and the quality of the education by how his or her students perform. Quality control is a part of every dietitian's job responsibility and is a managerial function.

Conceptual Skills

The manager performs a certain number of activities based on visualizing the larger picture beyond the technical aspects of his or her position. The ability to realistically anticipate the future, to plan and set goals, to provide direction in an organization, and to model professional behavior constitutes conceptual ability or skill.

Strategic Planning and Goal Setting

In general, strategic planning occurs at the upper levels of management as it requires data gathering and analysis; development of strategies, goals, and objectives, and implementation of action plans. However, professionals at all levels in an organization participate in data gathering and in setting short- and long-term goals. They are a part of the planning process to set direction and plans of action for the organization.

Some plans are general, such as the determination of values, mission, and vision statements. Others are more detailed and maybe developed at the supervisory level. If operational plans are short range, they are usually expected to occur within a year. Long-term plans extend beyond a year— sometimes beyond 10 years. The food and nutrition professional often contributes to both types of planning by conducting feasibility studies, cost-effectiveness studies, and quality-control measures.

Ethical Conduct

In dietetics, the *Code of Ethics for the Profession of Dietetics* is the guiding document to ethical practice. In any institution, the manager or leader assists in developing organization practices and policies that promote ethical practice. Such practices are established in purchasing, financial management, patient care issues, and information provided by patients and clients. The manager or leader sets the example for ethical behavior and integrity built on openness and trust.

Managing Change

Change occurs when there is dissatisfaction with things as they are and there is a desire to change them. Change may occur slowly or rapidly as in the event of sudden or unplanned circumstances. The leader who welcomes change and uses it to motivate and improve a department will be the most successful. When members of a unit work together to make changes, the efforts are usually rewarded by acceptance of the new procedure by all those affected. In contrast, if change is imposed by the leader without input from the other members, there is often resistance and slow acceptance.

Dietitians who counsel clients to make changes do not always meet with success. Time constraints and client expectations as well as motivations that differ from those of the dietitian are factors in the change process. Change models that take into consideration the complexities of behavior and one's approach to what it takes to help people change are often helpful. One approach is the use of goal setting in a way that the client being counseled is a part of the process and understands the expected outcome.[21]

The first step in initiating change is identifying the problem. One or more achievable goals for overcoming the problem are set next. In acting, persons typically mobilize their personal and social resources and identify barriers to reaching the goal. Self-monitoring and rewards provide additional motivation to attain the goal. The reward may be external, but an effective internal reward is one such as learning that leads to sustained performance and further goal setting.

Dietetics professionals constantly face change because of new developments in health care, organizational change, and shifts in management with a new mission and vision goals. Even environmental and political situations create change. When changes are viewed as opportunities, they are more likely to lead to positive results. The creative manage or leader helps create an atmosphere that welcomes and plans for this outcome.

Common Competencies for Healthcare Managers

The Healthcare Leadership Alliance is a consortium of six major professional organizations.[22] A study conducted by the alliance reported on the following five competencies common among practicing healthcare managers (**Figure 11-2**).

1. *Communication and relationship management*: The ability to communicate clearly and concisely with internal and external customers and to facilitate interactions with individuals and groups.

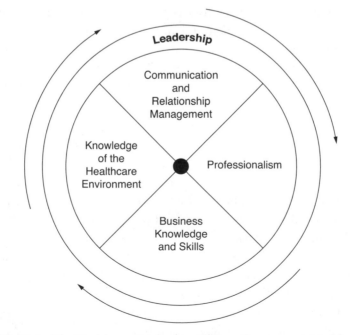

FIGURE 11-2. The Healthcare Leadership Alliance Competency Model

2. *Leadership*: The ability to inspire excellence, to create and attain shared vision, and to manage change.
3. *Professionalism*: The ability to align personal and organizational conduct with ethical and professional standards that include a responsibility to the patient and community, a service orientation, and a commitment to lifelong learning and improvement.
4. *Knowledge of the healthcare environment*: The demonstrated understanding of the healthcare system and the environment in which healthcare managers and providers function.
5. *Business skills and knowledge*: The ability to apply business principles, including systems thinking, in the healthcare environment.

MANAGEMENT IN PRACTICE

Alongside and complementing the traditional roles of management—planning, organizing, coordinating, controlling—are behavioral roles that might be described as functional improvement roles. For instance, by regularly reviewing and updating strategic plans, newer methods, organizational changes, and environmental changes can be readily incorporated into the plans. Issues such as disaster planning, recycling programs, and the green movement all impact the work unit and therefore require managerial decisions and planning. The policy manual should be viewed as a working document that is referred to often.

Doing more with less is almost a way of life in most institutions. This means that the manager needs to have a grasp of good business practices. Successful managers turn to strategies such as looking for ways to outsource beyond the department; reviewing all departmental procedures; and incorporating all possible technical assistance.

Personnel issues are without doubt one of the most time-consuming but critical parts of a manager's job. Motivating and inspiring is a large part of the job, which requires constant and effective communication, feedback on performance, and a conscious focus on cultural issues. Likewise, reviewing and updating training methods and materials can be an effective way of keeping personnel interested and motivated.

A focus on quality in every aspect of a food service system or clinical unit is a must in order to ensure acceptance by patients and clients. Even though quality is not easy to define, it is recognized—both when apparent and when lacking. The astute manager continually monitors performance of the unit by using customer surveys and informal feedback and by soliciting employee input. He or she regularly reviews all standards of ethical practice and ensures that they are fully understood and practiced by all in the organization. Ethical practices at all levels in a department create the environment in which an emphasis on quality is routine and ongoing.

The effective manager uses all available resources for continual improvement. Using the evidence-based library materials, networking with others in a practice group, and mentoring students and interns help keep the practitioner current. Further, the manager of the unit will benefit by ensuring that others in the work unit have continued education opportunities.

The management role is one that is multifaceted. It is one that requires technical know-how but just as importantly, people skills, as has been pointed out in the descriptions of managers' multiple roles.

SUMMARY

Managers and leaders possess many characteristics that are similar, but there are differences in roles and responsibilities. The skillful manager possesses human, technical, and conceptual abilities that permit him or her to accomplish work through coworkers and to attain goals. The leader may perform some or all of these same functions but will also inspire, motivate, and create a sense of unity and purpose. The dietitian, regardless of the area of practice, must perform managerial functions such as goal setting, communicating, team building, and managing resources. Many critical functions in the workplace will also require the dietitian to lead.

DEFINITIONS

Benchmarking. Comparing performance measures for the development of better methods and procedures.

Coach. A person who guides, inspires, and motivates.

Leadership. The qualities that allow an individual to influence the actions of others.

Management. The activities by which an organization functions.

Mentor. A person who teaches and guides by instructing, demonstrating, encouraging, and role modeling.

Resource management. The handling of money, equipment and supplies, or personnel essential to the administration of an organizational unit. *Strategic planning.* Long-range planning that involves data gathering, data analysis, development of goals and objectives, and action plans.

REFERENCES

1. Covey, S.R. *Principle-Centered Leadership.* (New York: Simon and Schuster, 1990).
2. Canter, D.D., K.L. Sauer, and C.W. Shanklin. "Management Is a Multifaceted Component Essential to the Skill Set of Successful Dietetics Practitioners." *J Acad Nutr Diet* 112, suppl. 2 (2012): S5.
3. Frank, G.C. *Community Nutrition: Applying Epidemiology to Contemporary Practice.* (Sudbury, MA: Jones and Bartlett, 2008).
4. Drucker, P.F. *Managing for the Future: The 1990s and Beyond.* (New York: Ruman Talley Books, Plume, 1992).
5. Cloud, H. In: Kaufman, M. *Nutrition in Promoting the Public's Health. Strategies, Principles, and Practice.* (Sudbury, MA: Jones and Bartlett, 2007), 537–549.
6. Leadership Institute, Accessed May 15, 2012, www.eatright.org
7. Gregoire, M.B., and S.W Arendt. "Leadership: Reflections Over the Past 100 Years." *J Am Diet Assoc* 104 (2004): 395–403.
8. Hunter, A.M.B., N.M. Lewis, and P.K. Ritter-Gooder. "Constructive Developmental Theory: An Alternative Approach to Leadership." *J Am Diet Assoc* 111 (2011): 1804–1808.
9. Coleman, E. "What Makes a Leader?" *Har Bus Rev* (November–December 1998): 23–32.
10. McLearney, A.S. "Using Leadership Development Programs to Improve Quality and Efficiency in Healthcare." *J Healthc Manag* 53, no. 5 (2008): 319–331.
11. Gould, R.S., and D. Canter. "Management Matters." *J Am Diet Assoc* 108 (2008): 1834–1836.
12. Canter, D.D., and M.F. Nettles. "Dietitians as Multidepartment Managers in Health Care Settings." *J Am Diet Assoc* 103 (2003): 237–240.
13. Brown, D. "Ways Dietitians of Different Generations Can Work Together." *J Am Diet Assoc* 103 (2003): 1461–1462.
14. Cant, R. "Constructions of Competence within Dietetics: Trust, Professionalism and Communications with Individual Clients." Journal Compilation 2009. *Diet Aust* (2009): 113–118.
15. Curtis, Elk, and R. O'Connell. "Essential Leadership Skills for Motivating and Developing Staff." *Nurs Manage* 18 (2011): 32–35.
16. Bartosek, C.B. In: Kaufman, M. *Nutrition in Promoting the Public Health: Strategies, Principles, and Practice.* (Sudbury, MA: Jones and Bartlett, 2007), 471.
17. McKnight, I.E.G., M.L. Dundas, and J.T. Girvan. "Dietetics Program Directors Areas of Practice." *J Am Diet Assoc* 102 (2002): 82–84.

18. Johnson, B.C., and J. Chambers. "Foodservice Benchmarking: Practices, Attitudes, and Beliefs of Foodservice Directors." *J Am Diet Assoc* 100 (2000): 175–180.
19. Weisberg, K. "Spirited Pioneer." *Foodservice Dir* (May 2007): 65–66.
20. Ward. B., D. Roger, C. Mueller, R. Touger-Decker, and K.L. Sauer. "Entry-Level Dietetics Practice Today: Results from the 2010 Commission on Dietetic Registration Entry-Level Dietetics Practice Audit." *J Am Diet Assoc* 111 (2011): 914–941.
21. Cullen, K.W., T. Baranowski, and S.P. Smith. "Using Goal setting as a Strategy for Dietary Behavior Change." *J Am Diet Assoc* 101 (2001): 562–565.
22. Steff, M.E. "Common Competencies for All Healthcare Managers: The Healthcare Leadership Alliance Model." *J Healthc Manage* 53 (2008): 360–373.

CHAPTER 12

The Dietitian as Educator

"Continuing education within the workforce must be coupled with lifelong learning to keep pace with advancements made within healthcare and technology."[1]

OUTLINE

- Introduction
- Educational Activities of Dietitians
- Learning to Teach
- Career Opportunities in Education
  - Elementary and Secondary Schools
  - Colleges and Universities
  - Medical and Dental Education
  - Nursing and Allied Health Nutrition Education
  - Industry-Based Education
  - Work-Site Nutrition Education
- Educator Roles
  - Mentor
  - Coach
  - Preceptor
  - Counselor
  - Communicator
- Types of Learning
  - Service Learning
  - Problem-Based Learning
  - Project-Based Learning
- Adults as Learners

INTRODUCTION

Dietitians sometimes reveal that they chose dietetics as a career in part because they did not view themselves as teachers. The reality, however, is that all dietitians are educators, most frequently in locations other than the classroom. The educational settings are as diverse as the careers in which dietitians work; the learners are individuals and groups of all ages. For example, the dietitian who works in clinical dietetics in a hospital or healthcare center teaches patients, families, and allied health personnel. A dietitian in food service management teaches and trains food service personnel and may teach personnel in other departments. Dietitians in business or private practice may teach patients, other personnel, and the public. In all areas of practice, the dietitian may also teach dietetic interns and dietetic technician students.

The educator role is one of the most important a dietitian fulfills. Knowledge of subject matter is attained by the professional through academic preparation in a degree program and practical experience in a supervised practice program. Added to this knowledge is an understanding of how to teach effectively and how people learn. Observation of other educators, continuing education, and professional experience, as well as practice, lead to expertise as an educator.

Dietitians need to possess several skills related to teaching. These include verbal and nonverbal communications, speaking to groups, behavior modification and motivation, principles of learning, teaching techniques, and knowledge about how to work with groups. These skills can be learned and improved the more they are practiced.

Dietitians in education typically affiliate with one of the three following dietetic practice groups: Nutrition Education for the Public, Nutrition Educators of Health Professionals, or Dietetic Educators of Practitioners.

EDUCATIONAL ACTIVITIES OF DIETITIANS

The 2010 audit of practice areas by the Commission on Dietetic Registration (CDR)[2] indicated the kinds of educational activities performed by entry-level dietitians and dietetic technicians. The activities are shown in **Table 12-1**.

Table 12-1. Educational Activities Performed by Entry-Level Dietitians and Dietetic Technicians

Activity	RD Percent	DTR Percent
Assess learning needs of patients/clients, employees, students	90	73
Develop instructional materials for individuals and groups	81	58
Teach classes or laboratories	48	38
Evaluate learner knowledge and performance	64	48
Supervise students or precept interns	55	32
Provide health-promotion or risk-reduction programs to population groups	21	12
Distribute nutrition information through the media	17	6
Design individual courses or seminars for patients, clients, employees, students		51
Design group-related courses for educational institutions	16	0
Evaluate educational programs	23	0
Design services to meet nutrition-related needs of populations	19	0

Source: This article was published in the Journal of the American Dietetic Association, 92(12), Roach, et al, "Improving Dietitians' Teaching Skills," pp. 1749–1757, Copyright Elsevier (2001).

LEARNING TO TEACH

Teaching skills are developed when the educator follows a process that will result in an effective outcome; i.e., the learner is a participant in the process and acquires new knowledge. Depending on the type of teaching session—formal as in a classroom or informal as in the workplace—the process may involve a very structured plan that follows specific steps or a more flexible plan with input from learners.

The steps in the process are the following:

1. The assessment of learner needs
2. The development of performance objectives
3. The instructional strategy including content and delivery method
4. Preparation of instructional materials
5. Evaluation or follow-up of the learning session

The steps may be shortened or compressed in informal teaching situations; nevertheless, thought should be given to each of the steps whether in a one-on-one session or in group sessions. In the first step, the assessment of learner needs is the basis for planning a teaching session. This may be determined from practical experience and observation of job performance, a change in organizational needs, a job change, or whether it is new information or a reinforcement of the learner's understanding of information presented earlier. Having one or more objectives in mind gives focus to the teaching session and provides a reference later as to the effectiveness of the lesson.

The content of the lesson and the way the material is to be presented require advance planning along with the determination of teaching aids needed. The content and the way it is presented can vary widely, and the instructor makes choices about both based on the size of the group, the makeup of the group, and the needs of the group. An experienced teacher knows the type of presentation that is most effective in certain situations and uses this in planning the lesson.

The final step is to assess what the learner has learned and therefore the success of the teaching session. This may occur at the time of a teaching session or in follow-up sessions and may be by observation, questioning, or testing.

Online education is an increasingly popular method of presenting educational material, and it should be noted that the same process is followed when designing this type of instruction.[3]

Several observations that will assist the instructor in planning and conducting learning sessions are the following:

1. Learners hear and process information in individual ways. Repetition and variety in presentation will often mean better reception.
2. Introduce key points early in the session and repeat as necessary.
3. The learners' previous knowledge influences what they learn in a new situation.
4. Present new information in small amounts at a time. Illustrate new concepts and facts with examples and easily understood terminology related to the workplace or class subject.
5. Encourage active learning by participation of the learner. Encourage questions, give time for discussion, and give assignments for future sessions or follow-up if applicable.

CAREER OPPORTUNITIES IN EDUCATION

While all dietitians will perform at times in teaching roles in whatever area of practice they are employed, there is a diversity of employment areas in education that dietitians may pursue. These are discussed in the following sections.

Elementary and Secondary Schools

School-based nutrition education is incorporated into health and science classes in primary, middle, and high schools. A dietitian who teaches at these levels must meet state teacher training and certification requirements. Generally, those who teach grades K–12 have responsibilities that extend well beyond food, nutrition, and health.

Some state departments of education have nutrition education and training sections that often employ registered dietitians who have advanced degrees in education. Such positions include creating curricula to integrate nutrition with other subjects, developing teaching materials, identifying instructional resources, and training teachers to deliver nutrition education.

Job opportunities for dietitians in child nutrition programs affect dietitians from the lunchroom to the classroom. School-based health centers—rapidly growing models for the delivery of comprehensive primary health care in elementary, middle, and high schools—afford another opportunity for dietitians interested in working with children and adolescents.[4] There is also a need in these school-based centers for dietitians certified by the CDR for weight management of children and adolescents.[5]

Colleges and Universities

There are teaching opportunities for dietitians in culinary institutes, technical schools, and 2- or 4-year colleges. Such positions are often associated with programs for chefs, food service supervisors, dietetic technicians, dietary managers, entry-level dietitians, and hospitality managers. The emphasis is on teaching in the classroom, laboratory, or practice setting. Course responsibilities may include food preparation and food science, basic and applied nutrition, meal management, cultural food practices, food service management and equipment, nutrition assessment and therapy, nutrition counseling and education, and community nutrition.

University faculty roles are quite varied. In addition to their teaching responsibilities, university faculty are required to conduct research and provide service within the institution, community, or profession. They advise students on academic choices and research, serve on committees, consult with community groups, share their expertise with the media and the public, and provide departmental and university leadership for nutrition-related initiatives.

Higher education can include teaching other groups of students. For example, some institutions offer nutrition courses for nondietetics majors to fulfill requirements for general education, teacher certification, or health and physical education. Programs in the allied health professions may include nutrition courses. Dietitians can teach courses in nutritional anthropology or epidemiology, often included as part of the master's degree in public health programs.

Medical and Dental Education

Some graduate-trained dietitians are engaged in medical and dental education. Such a role requires assertiveness and creativity to convince administrators of the unique contributions that dietitians have to offer in medical and dental education. For an emphasis on prevention and health promotion, nutrition is a required component, and dietitians are the best qualified persons to provide this education. An in-depth knowledge of nutrition science and medical nutrition therapy is required. Additionally, medical and dental nutrition educators must possess leadership ability, self-direction, strong communication skills, conceptual thinking skills, time management techniques, and flexibility.

Nutrition education can occur at any level of a medical or dental curriculum. It may consist of nutrition science with clinical application during the first 2 years while basic information is the major part of the curriculum. As students enter the clinical part of their program, sample meals featuring special diets are often effective teaching tools. Nutrition rounds and seminars can be incorporated when students are in residencies. Practicing dietitians can be involved in problem-based learning as an effective way to make nutrition relevant for future medical practice.

Nursing and Allied Health Nutrition Education

Nutrition services are often provided by nondietitians, depending on the practice setting and contributions of various health professionals. For example, nurses regularly monitor food intake, evaluate laboratory values indicative of nutritional status, and give patients nutritional advice. Dental hygienists and health educators often screen for health or nutritional problems and provide education and intervention. All health professionals should understand the role nutrition plays in wellness and disease prevention, and they need training on appropriate interventions. Nutrition is included in the curriculum for nurses' training programs, and dietitians often teach the courses.

Industry-Based Education

Companies that manufacture medical nutrition products often employ dietitians to provide technical and clinical information to the sales force and to other personnel, including clinicians, retail pharmacists, and educators of healthcare professionals. Dietitians may educate via telephone, webinars, written correspondence, electronic mail, and by personal visits. They may participate in developing video, audio, and slide programs; technical monographs; newsletters; brochures; and professional and patient education publications on topics of medical nutrition therapy.

Companies that manufacture institutional equipment, food products, supplemental products such as high-protein and other preparations for tube feedings, infant formula, and supplements for nutritional additives may also employ dietitians to help promote and demonstrate the use of the products.

Personal characteristics and skills necessary for success in industry-based education include technical and professional proficiency, ability to critically and objectively analyze issues, attention to detail, high work standards, skill in written and oral communications, adaptability, and ability to tolerate stress. Clearly, such positions require a proficiency in nutritional science, practitioner experience, conceptual and analytic skills, altruistic values, and a service ethic.

Work-Site Nutrition Education

As increased attention is given to the role of nutrition in health and disease prevention, more opportunities for dietitians will open in work-site wellness programs. These work sites may include manufacturing plants, insurance companies, and service organizations. Some of these positions will focus entirely on nutrition education and may include screening for nutritional risk, program development, leading classes and demonstrations, creating exhibits and displays, and evaluating the effectiveness of nutrition education initiatives. Dietitians in these positions may provide valuable experience for dietetic interns or other students as well.

Work-site education opportunities can also include coordinators of training in large dietetics departments or at the regional level of contract food and nutrition service companies. Dietitians in such roles may oversee a dietetic internship, coordinate in-service training for food service and other personnel, and direct training for students from affiliating programs. Individuals with the appropriate background may be promoted to director of training and development at the institutional or corporate level.

EDUCATOR ROLES

As shown in the CDR audit of dietetics practice, dietitians participate in many activities in which they teach employees, patients, allied health professionals, students, and consumers. A variety of approaches are used to reach the desired audience, all of which involve communication. Verbal interaction and nonverbal cues enter into the effectiveness of the message, and the skilled educator takes into account the best way to communicate with the learner. Several of the roles by which dietitians interact with learners are discussed in the following section.

Mentor

A mentor is a person who may teach verbally, by demonstration of particular activities or skills, by role modeling, or by a combination of these approaches. The mentoring relationship is a shared experience between a teacher and a learner. A mentor may be one's peer, an instructor, a trusted advisor, or anyone more skilled—think of the teenager who helps a parent or grandparent become computer literate. The mentor may also be described as a tutor in that one-on-one teaching is the method used.

A successful statewide mentoring program for dietitians in California resulted in a positive feedback from both mentors and those mentored.[6] In the program, district training was conducted. The most meaningful outcomes of the training were the following:

- Positive feedback from those mentored
- Help with career change
- Networking and finding mentors through interactions
- The opportunity to provide support to RDs
- Connection of RDs with those who desire to learn new skills
- Beneficial new areas of opportunity
- Informal contacts with students
- Assistance for prospective RDs in education plans for RD certification
- Resources available to those interested in the mentoring process

The Nutrition Entrepreneurs practice group conducts a mentorship program aimed toward matching volunteer mentors with other members who need guidance to make their vision a reality.[7] The mentor program offers rewards for both mentors and those mentored.

Coach

A coach is one who inspires and motivates others. Coaching is sometimes described as the role assumed with individuals who are already achieving at a high level and is simply positive feedback for continued high performance. The coaching role is effective when involvement and trust are created, expectations are clarified, performance is acknowledged, actions are challenged, and achievement is rewarded. The football coach is the classic example of one who performs all these functions in the expectation of having a winning team.

Coaching is similar to reflective teaching in that the teacher may demonstrate a new procedure or piece of information, and the learner repeats the procedure. The coach responds with advice, criticism, explanation, description, or further demonstration. The learner reflects and compares the new information to his or her previous knowledge and acts accordingly.

Preceptor

The preceptor is one who provides direction and instruction, supervised performance, and evaluates learners in applied practice. The dietitian who oversees a dietetic intern in supervised practice has the title of preceptor. A preceptor must have good interpersonal and time-management skills as well as subject-matter competence as a skilled practitioner. Preceptors are essential in dietetics education and to the future of dietetic practice. They should consult and follow the *Standards of Practice and Standards of Professional Performance for Registered Dietitians (Generalist, Specialty, Advanced) in Education of Dietetics Practitioners* developed by the American Dietetic Association and educators to guide their practice.[8]

Many benefits are realized by both the preceptor and the student as well as the department or institution providing experiences for the student. Among the benefits for preceptors observed in one study were assisting students with application of knowledge and expertise, gaining personal satisfaction, observing students' growth from novice to practitioner, and stimulating ongoing interest in the profession.[9] Students gained valuable knowledge from the example set by experienced professionals and were guided to levels of achievement that allowed them to assume entry-level positions well prepared.

Descriptions of the various roles as perceived by the teacher, preceptor/ teacher, preceptor/mentor, and mentor are shown in **Table 12-2**.

Counselor

Counseling is a process of listening, accepting, clarifying, and helping clients or students form conclusions and develop plans of action. The process is guided toward helping individuals learn about their needs and about methods of coping with them.

Motivational interviewing is defined as a way of helping others bring about behavior change, such as curbing addictive behaviors.[10] This technique was used in a study that led to increased fruit and vegetable intake

Table 12-2. Preceptor Roles

	Teacher	Preceptor/Teacher	Preceptor	Preceptor/Mentor	Mentor
View of intern	View intern as a student[a]		View intern as a prospective coworker[b]		View intern as a colleague[b]
Conceptual focus	Focus on discipline-based learning[b]		Focus on practice-based learning[a]		Focus on personal development[b]
Prior knowledge		Assess intern's prior content knowledge[c]		Assume intern has necessary content knowledge[b]	
Theory/practice	Teach basic subject matter[b]		Demonstrate the incorporation of theory in practice[a]		Identify unwritten workplace policies and practices[b]
Learning experiences	Arrange useful learning experiences to help intern achieve objectives[a]		Suggest useful learning experiences to help intern achieve learning objectives[a]		Encourage intern to determine learning experiences to achieve objectives[c]
Ethical concerns		Discuss potential ethical issues[c]		Identify actual ethical concerns[b]	
Strengths-weaknesses	Identify intern's strengths and weaknesses[a]			Help intern become aware of strengths and weaknesses[a]	

(continues)

Table 12-2. Preceptor Roles *(continued)*

	Teacher	Preceptor/Teacher	Preceptor	Preceptor/Mentor	Mentor
Progress evaluation	Provide intern with an evaluation of academic progress[c]			Provide intern with an evaluation of professional progress[a]	
Intern self-evaluation			Identify usefulness of self-evaluation[c]		Strongly encourage intern to participate in self-evaluation[c]
Role model	View yourself as an academic role model[a]		View yourself as a professional role model[a]		View yourself as a personal role model[a]
Duration of relationship		Recognize relationship with intern is limited[a]			View the relationship with the intern as indefinite[b]

Columns represent the categorical descriptions for each role. Rows represent the functions/elements that relate to the supervised practice experience. [a]Practices preceptors indicated they "frequently" execute and do not want to change. [b]Practices preceptors executed in varying degrees from frequently or occasionally to seldom/never, but do not want to change. [c]Practice preceptors believed they should do more often.

Source: Reprinted from Journal of the American Dietetic Association 102, Number 7 (July 2002), Wilson, M.A. "Dietetic Preceptors Perceive Their Role to Include a Variety of Elements," 969, Copyright 2002, with permission from Elsevier.

by African Americans.[11] This type of counseling is also described as a directive, client-centered style for eliciting behavior change by helping clients explore and resolve ambivalence.

A cognitive interview technique is sometimes used to assist in understanding how audiences or individuals process information. Respondents are led through a survey or message and asked to respond with their thoughts, feelings, or ideas that come to mind. With this information, better messages are formed and valuation tools are targeted.[12]

Patient-centered counseling facilitates change by assessing patients' needs and tailoring the intervention to the patient's stage in the process of change, personal goals, and unique challenges.[13] Four steps are followed: assessment, advising, assisting, and follow-up. In step one, the dietitian-counselor asks questions to determine present behaviors. Open-ended questions will help gain this information. (See **Table 12-3** for examples). In step two, advisement based on the assessment is given toward helping the person make changes. Assisting, in step three, involves giving motivational statements and encouragement. Goals and specific skills such as self-monitoring and problem-solving will also be discussed. In the final step, follow-up toward maintaining dietary change will be presented and attainment of earlier goals discussed. Further help will also be provided.

Communicator

Effective communication is of utmost importance in all areas of dietetics, and almost any job description will include the need to communicate at all levels in an organization as well as with individuals. Professionals who develop verbal and written skills, along with listening skills, establish stronger relationships with clients, patients, and staff.

There are, at a minimum, seven components of the communication process. Seven of the components are as follows:

1. *Source.* The source is the starting point for information exchange.
2. *Message.* The message is the idea or information transmitted verbally or nonverbally.
3. *Channel.* The channel is the pathway for messages between the sender and the receiver.
4. *Receiver.* The receiver takes in the message, assigns meaning, interprets, and responds to the message.

Table 12-3. A Model for Open-Ended Questioning

Questions for Assessing Stage of Change and Motivation

How do you feel about your current diet?

What problems have you had because of your diet?

What would you like to change about your diet now?

Why would you like to change your diet now?

What concerns do you have about changing your diet now?

What reasons might you have to want to maintain your current diet?

What would motivate you to maintain your current diet?

Questions for Assessing Past Experiences with Dietary Change

What changes have you made to your diet? How long did you maintain the changes? If so, for how long? If not, how long did you maintain the change?

How did you make changes in your diet? What helped?

What difficulties did you encounter? How did you handle them?

Questions about Anticipated Challenges or Barriers to Change

What could get in your way of attaining your goal?

What situations will make it hardest for you to achieve your goal?

What other situations might make it difficult for you to maintain your change?

Questions about Strategies to Cope with Challenges or Barriers to Change

What could you do when you face this challenge?

What else could you do in the face of this challenge or barrier?

Who could help you cope with this challenge? How?

What has been helpful in the past to deal with this barrier?

Questions for Goal Setting

What are you willing to change in your diet now?

When? How often will you do this?

Where will you do it?

What will you have to do in advance to ensure that you are able to make and maintain this change?

How confident are you of your ability to make and maintain this change?

Questions for Follow-Up

How did you do with your plan?

What helped you stay on target?

What difficulties did you encounter?

Questions for Assessing Lapse and Relapse

What made it difficult for you to stay with your plan?

How did you feel after that?

What else could you have done to stay on track?

What would you like to do now?

Source: Reprinted from Journal of the American Dietetic Association 101, Number 3 (March 2001), Rosal, M.C., C.B. Ebbeling, I. Lofgren, J.K. Ockene, I.S. Ockene, and J.R. Hebert. "Facilitating Dietary Change: The Patient-Centered Counseling Model," 333, Copyright 2001, with permission from Elsevier.

5. *Feedback.* Feedback refers to the response from the receiver to the sender.
6. *Environment.* The environment is the context in which the message occurs, such as physical surroundings and cultural, historic, or attitudinal factors.
7. *Noise.* Noise is any aural, visual, or internal factor that can distract from the meaning of the message.

The communication methods that ensure messages are received need to be carefully selected. Professionals who provide nutrition information to the public will choose methods such as television, Internet, or printed materials. The development of dietary guidance messages through the use of focus groups and surveys of consumers is described by Borra.[14] In the consumer message development model (**Figure 12-1**), the issues are defined, the message developed and assessed, then fine tuned and validated.

Today, while the use of e-mail, voice mail, and other social media are efficient, it should be emphasized that face-to-face communication is still important in many situations.[15] Human contact, especially in direct contact with patients, is the most reliable way of assuring the message is received because interaction can occur at the same time and reaction to the message assessed.

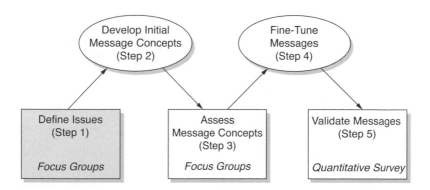

FIGURE 12-1. The Consumer Message Development Model.

Source: Reprinted from Journal of the American Dietetic Association 101, Number 6 (June 2001, Borra, S., L. Kelly, M. Tuttle, and K. Neville. "Developing Actionable Dietary Guidance Messages: Dietary Fat as a Case Study," 679, Copyright 2001, with permission from Elsevier.

In a study to determine the best means of communicating nutrition education for elderly adults, several factors were found to be successful.[16] They included limiting educational messages to one or two, reinforcing and personalizing messages, providing purposeful activities and incentives, providing access to health professionals, and using behavior change. A model was developed showing these elements (**Figure 12-2**).

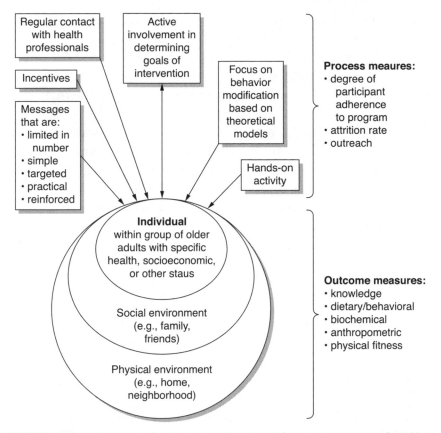

FIGURE 12-2. A Framework for Designing a Nutrition Education Intervention for Older Adults.

Source: Reprinted from Journal of the American Dietetic Association 104, Number 1 (January 2004), Sayhoun, N.R., C.A. Pratt, and A. Anderson. "Evaluation of Nutrition Education Interventions for Older Adults: A Proposed Framework," 66, Copyright 2004, with permission from Elsevier.

TYPES OF LEARNING

Education programs are based on learning outcomes or categories of learning, described as domains of learning. One classification, often used in education, describes five types of learning outcomes or skills as follows[17]:

1. *Psychomotor skills.* The learner acquires motor skills along with the know-how to perform tasks.
2. *Intellectual skills.* Information-processing skills allow the learner to perform a new activity.
3. *Verbal processing skills.* The learner is able to provide information through stating, listing, or describing something.
4. *Attitudinal skills.* The learner makes choices or decisions to act in certain ways. These may include long-term goals that determine a person's ability to perform psychomotor or other skills.
5. *Cognitive skills.* The learner has attained abstract strategies to become self-directed through the use of intellectual skills.

Another so-called index of learning styles[18] describes the following eight types of learning:

1. *Active.* An active learner likes trying things out and enjoys working in groups.
2. *Reflective.* A reflective learner thinks things through; he or she prefers working alone or with one or two partners.
3. *Sensing.* A sensing learner is concrete, practical, and oriented towards facts and procedures.
4. *Intuitive.* An intuitive learner is conceptual, innovative, and oriented toward theories and underling meanings.
5. *Visual.* A visual learner prefers visual representations or presented material.
6. *Verbal.* A verbal learner prefers written and spoken explanations.
7. *Sequential.* A sequential learner undertakes a linear thinking process and prefers learning in incremental steps.
8. *Global.* A global learner undertakes a holistic thinking process and prefers to learn in large steps.

Education through the use of methods that involve the learner in an active, participatory way can lead to very effective outcomes.

Internships are examples of service learning. Problem-based learning is the method by which a student discovers new knowledge through individual learning in solving a problem. Project-based learning, similar to problem-based, is the method in which learner involvement is guided by an instructor. These three types of learning are described in the following sections.

Service Learning

Service learning is the type of educational experience that combines explicit academic learning with service.[19] In many professions, combining classroom study and community learning experiences is a way of enhancing and retaining learning. In dietetics, the internship is an example because it combines practice with instruction. Another example is the college class that places students in a community site such as a school or elderly nutrition program for experiences that are a part of the course requirements. Seeing and experiencing nutrition applied in specific community programs makes subject matter come alive and leads to a better understanding of the value and need of community service.

Problem-Based Learning

A method often used in medical and business schools, problem-based learning requires students to work through problems to find answers to real-life situations. This provides a context for students to learn critical thinking and problem-solving skills and to acquire knowledge of the essential concepts of a course of study.[20] In this method, students are presented a problem and organized into groups to discuss the problem. Students pose questions and rank the learning issues generated in the session. Students and the instructor discuss the resources needed to research the learning issues. Students then summarize their knowledge and connect the new concepts to older ones and define new learning issues as they progress through the problem. The benefit is that students recognize that learning is an ongoing process with new learning issues to be explored.

The role of the instructor is to guide, probe, and support students' initiatives. When faculty incorporate problem-based learning into classes, they empower students to take a responsible role in their learning. As a result, faculty must be ready to yield some authority to their students.

Project-Based Learning

Similar to problem-based learning, project-based learning is a form of instruction that places emphasis on the students' involvement in working through job-related situations. It is described as a long-term, problem-focused, meaningful unit of instruction that integrates concepts from a number of disciplines. An example might be the design of a kitchen layout using work flow, equipment, and production schedules. Both teacher and student receive support in fulfilling their roles, the teacher as facilitator and shepherd of projects, and the student by participating in a worthwhile project. A project-based learning support system that supports learning through a computer-mediated interface using learner-centered software has been described.[21] This type of learning is useful in simulations or when students share a concentrated experience. New tools and structures are often needed to support the effectiveness of this type of learning, but it provides good results amid complex and challenging projects.

ADULTS AS LEARNERS

Conducting learning sessions for adults is different from teaching younger people. Dietitians need to be aware of the differences in order to adapt their teaching for the best learning outcomes. Adult learners, for example, have backgrounds of experience they bring to new learning situations and they are usually independent and self-directed. They may prefer to work alone or in small groups. Participating in activities and solving problems are typical preferences for learning styles as they may have immediate need for the information. Adults are often motivated by factors such as the need for an educational undertaking for economic or professional advancement reasons, a desire to learn new material, and for personal satisfaction. Even health reasons may factor into adult choices with the research showing that mental capacity is more readily maintained when the mind continues to be used throughout life.

TEACHING GROUPS AND TEAMS

Groups of people usually act in ways that are different than when they are in a one-on-one learning situation. *Group dynamics* is a term often applied to this behavior because it describes how members relate to each other, how they communicate among themselves, and how they work as a group. The teacher or leader of the group needs to understand how these dynamics can affect the learning process and the ways the educational message needs to be delivered.

Groups function best when all members participate because information is more likely to be shared and understood as new ideas, questions, clarifications, etc., occur. All group members need to understand the purpose and expected outcomes of the learning situation, and the leader has the responsibility to make sure this is clear at the outset of the lesson. When disagreements or tension arise in the group, the leader should be prepared to change the subject or take a time-out or use some other technique to get the group back on track. Giving support, encouraging discussion, and including all the group members in active participation helps assure the session will accomplish its goals.

While teams are focused as a work group, many of the same characteristics as evidenced in groups will also appear. Teams may be formed in order to accomplish more through the combined efforts and expertise of individual members. Participation in teams, however, requires that members understand their role and the expectations for the group.

When teams are formed, members may be uncertain of their role and will depend on a leader to guide them into a team role. There may be conflict as team members clarify the team's goals. The leader then needs to redirect the energies of the team by encouraging open communication. As relationships become cohesive, the team functions as a unit and develops patterns of communication and behavior. The leader facilitates decision making and problem solving. The team members find ways of handling conflict, and methods that become standards for evaluating team performance therefore develop.

SUMMARY

The role of educator is one of the most important of those performed by the dietitian and dietetic technician. To be an effective educational leader, the professional must have a working knowledge of the education process by assessing learners' basic knowledge, setting learning goals, planning learning content and delivery methods, and evaluating the outcomes of the learning.

The dietitian may function in a number of educator roles, including that of mentor, coach, preceptor, or counselor. The effective teacher in any of these roles is skilled in communications and has the qualities of a leader in understanding individuals and groups and fostering productive learning situations.

DEFINITIONS

Assessment. The process of evaluating actions or conditions on which to base additional activity.

Cognitive skills. The application of intellectual capabilities to accomplish objectives.

Education. The systematic instruction and training designed to impart knowledge and develop a skill.

Instruction. The activity by which knowledge or teaching is imparted.

Psychomotor skills. The ability to perform physical tasks based on knowing or thinking.

Training. Actions by which persons are brought to a desired standard of efficiency or behavior by instruction and practice.

REFERENCES

1. Boyce, B. "2011 Future Connections Summit on Dietetic Practice, Credentialing, and Education: Summary of Presentations on Shaping the Future of the Dietetic Profession." *J Am Diet Assoc* 111 (2011): 1591–1599.
2. Ward, B., D. Rogers, C. Mueller, R. Touger-Decker, and K.L. Sauer. "Entry-Level Dietetics Practice Today: Results from the 2010 Commission of Dietetic Registration Entry-Level Dietetics Practice Audit." *J Am Diet Assoc* 111 (2011): 914–941.
3. Sandon, L. "A System for Designing Effective Online Education." *J Am Diet Assoc* 107 (2007): 1305–1306.
4. "Position of the American Dietetic Association, School Nutrition Association, and Society for Nutrition Education: Comprehensive School Nutrition Services." *J Am Diet Assoc* 110 (2010): 1738–1749.
5. American Dietetic Association. "Certificate of Training in Childhood and Adolescent Weight Management." Accessed April 15, 2012, www.eatright.org
6. Schatz, P.E., T.J. Bush-Zurn, C. Aresa, and K.C. Freeman. "California's Professional Mentoring Program: How to Develop a Statewide Mentoring Program." *J Am Diet Assoc* 103 (2003): 73–76.
7. Bitzer, R., Nutrition Entrepreneurs Practice Group. "Mentor Program." *Ventures* XXV, no. 4 (2009): 11.

8. Anderson, J.A., K. Kennedy-Hagen, M.R. Stieber, D.S. Hollingsworth, K. Kattelman, C.L. Stein-Arnold, and B.M. Egan. "Dietetics Educators of Practitioners and Dietetic Association Standards of Professional Performance for Registered Dietitians (Generalist, Specialty/Advanced) in Education of Dietetics Practitioners." *J Am Diet Assoc* 109 (2009): 747–754.

9. Marincic, P.Z., and E.E. Francfort. "Supervised Program Preceptors' Perceptions of Rewards, Benefits, Support, and Commitment to the Preceptor Role." *J Am Diet Assoc* 102 (2002): 543–545.

10. Thorpe, M. "Motivational Interviewing and Dietary Behavior Change." *J Am Diet Assoc* 103 (2003): 150–151.

11. Resicow, K., A. Jackson, T. Wang, F. McCarty, W.W. Dudley, and T. Baranowski. "A Motivational Interviewing Intervention to Increase Fruit and Vegetable Intake Through Black Churches; Results of the Eat for Life Trial." *Am J Pub Health* 91 (2001): 1686–1693.

12. Carbone, E.T., M.K. Campbell, and L. Honess-Morreal. "Use of Cognitive Interview Techniques in the Development of Nutrition Surveys and Interactive Messages for Low-Income Populations." *J Am Diet Assoc* 102 (2002): 690–696.

13. Rosal, M.C., C.B. Ebbeling, I. Lofgren, J.K. Ockene, I.S. Ockene, and J.R. Hebert. "Facilitating Dietary Change: The Patient-Centered Counseling Model." *J Am Diet Assoc* 101 (2001): 332–341.

14. Borra, S., L. Kelly, M. Tuttle, and K. Neville. "Developing Actionable Dietary Guidance Messages: Dietary Fat as a Case Study." *J Am Diet Assoc* 101 (2001): 678–684.

15. Hallowell, E.M. "The Human Moment at Work." *Harvard Bus Review* (January–February 1999): 1–8.

16. Sayhoun, N.R., C.A. Oratt, and A. Anderson. "Evaluation of Nutrition Education Interventions for Older Adults: A Proposed Framework." *J Am Diet Assoc* 104 (2001): 58–69.

17. Gagne, R.M. *Instructional Technology: Foundations.* (Hillsdale, NJ: Lawrence Erlbaum Associates, 1987), p. 25.

18. Palermo, C., K.Z. Walker, T. Brown, and M. Zogi. "How Dietetics Students Like to Learn: Implications for Curriculum Planners." Dietitians Association of Australia. *J Compilation* (2009).

19. Kim, Y., and A. Canfield. "How to Develop a Service Learning Program in Dietetics Education." *J Am Diet Assoc* 102 (2002): 174–176.

20. Dietetic Educators of Practitioners Practice Group. "Problem-Based Learning: Preparing Students to Succeed in the 21st Century." *DEP Line* 17, no. 3 (1998): 1–5.

21. Laffey, J., T. Tupper, D. Musser, and J. Wedman. "A Computer-Mediated Support for Project-Based Learning." *Technology Research and Development* 46, no. 1 (1998): 73–86.

CHAPTER 13

The Dietitian as Researcher

"Research is the foundation of our profession."[1]

INTRODUCTION

Many dietitians conduct research as a part of their work. This is especially true for dietitians who specialize in nutrition support, pediatrics, renal dietetics, oncology, AIDS, or diabetes. These dietitians and those in all other areas of practice use research in various ways, may critique research, and collect research data for professional reference as needed. All dietitians are encouraged to perform or collect data for outcome research studies to demonstrate the effectiveness of medical nutrition therapy and/or the quality and acceptance of the services performed. In the clinical setting, dietitians may collaborate with physicians who are conducting nutrition-related studies, and even though they may not call themselves researchers, they are in fact participating in research and are critical to the process.

With the increasing emphasis on research in the Academy of Nutrition and Dietetics and in the profession generally, many dietitians are incorporating research studies into their practice. In part, there is a sense that more applied research studies are needed as more basic, laboratory-oriented research does not always meet the needs of everyday practice. To this end, a member network called the Dietetics Practice-Based Research Network (DPBRN) has been formed.[2] The network is open to all who are interested in addressing questions encountered in practice and to continually improve the delivery of food and nutrition services.

The DPBRN brings practitioners and researchers together to identify research that is needed in practice settings, to design significant research to obtain funding, and to carry the research into real-life practice. The focus of the research conducted by members is on studies that can be immediately incorporated into practice. Professionals who lack the time, money, or expertise to conduct research on their own find this group activity presents an opportunity to benefit from research by answering questions and keeping abreast of new information and to improve their practice.

IMPORTANCE OF RESEARCH IN DIETETICS

"Research represents the future for dietetics; it is the foundation for our credibility, our recognition, and our professional respect. Without research, we cannot properly educate or advocate, nor would we have the credibility in either endeavor."[3] All professions continually reshape themselves to meet ever-changing needs in society and research is essential for these changes and advancements to take place. Not only do dietitians need to engage in research to gain knowledge and define new modes of therapy and new techniques in all areas of practice, they also need to take a scholarly approach to everyday practice. Many practicing dietitians have an image of research as overwhelming or irrelevant, when in fact the reality is dramatically different. There are a number of exciting and relatively large ways for practicing dietitians to become involved with research, ranging from simply learning more about dietetics-related research, to evaluating research findings to make evidence-based decisions in work settings, to actually taking part in scientific projects.[4]

Employers of dietitians and those using dietetic services need to be assured that the services they are using are supported by research. Research is the basis for education because it drives the core knowledge and competencies and is used in setting public policy. The ability to conduct and use research further allows professionals to be recognized by the public as a valued and credible source of scientific nutrition information.

THE RESEARCH PHILOSOPHY OF THE ACADEMY

The research philosophy of the profession is the following:

> The Academy of Nutrition and Dietetics believes that research is the foundation of the profession, providing the basis for practice, education, and policy. Dietetics is the integration and application of principles derived from the sciences of nutrition, biochemistry, physiology, food management, and behavioral and social sciences to achieve and maintain people's health; therefore dietetics research is a dynamic collaborative and assimilative endeavor. This research is broad in scope, ranging from basic to applied practice research.[5]

The academy uses research as the basis of decisions, policy, and communication in a variety of roles. The roles include the following:

- *Advocate*. Federal and nongovernmental agencies, organizations, and individuals who can support the academy's research agenda.
- *Facilitator*. Targets key research questions and facilitates a successful process to answer the questions.

- *Convener.* Brings together scientists and practitioners from various disciplines to explore new approaches in solving research questions.
- *Funder.* Prepares, disseminates, and funds research proposals on key research questions important to the profession.
- *Educator.* Develops professional opportunities for members to enhance their knowledge and use of research.
- *Disseminator.* Distributes research results to members and the public through publications, work sites, and print and electronic media.

THE ACADEMY'S RESEARCH PRIORITIES

The Research Committee

The Research Committee of the academy, reporting to the board of directors and the house of delegates, sets the research agenda for the academy. In this capacity, the committee develops, maintains, and evaluates the research priorities.[6] The academy's statement of purpose emphasizes research: "The Academy is committed to improving the nation's health and advancing the profession of dietetics through research, education, and advocacy."[7] Two specific strategies to help reach these goals are to equip members to use research in their work, and to provide research and resources that can be translated into evidence-based practice.

The research committee identifies the priority research as core research and dietetics-specific or applied research. The core priorities are:

1. Nutrition and lifestyle-change intervention to prevent or treat obesity and chronic diseases
2. A safe, secure, and sustainable food supply
3. Nutrients and systems

The dietetics-specific priorities are:

1. Nutrition care process and health outcome measures
2. Reimbursement of dietetic services
3. Dietetics education and retention

Funding for approved projects comes from the academy foundation and other academy-affiliated groups, from governmental agencies, and from the food and nutrition industry. A tool kit that provides a lesson tutorial, practice suggestions, and resources for conducting research is available from the headquarters office.

Figure 13-1 illustrates the research priorities of the academy and the interaction between practice, education, and policy. Two major areas of research are identified: core research and dietetics-specific or applied research. The types of research considered priorities and that are emphasized in funding opportunities are shown in **Table 13-1**.

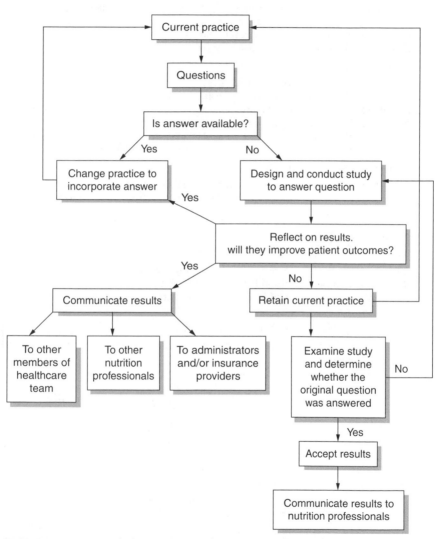

FIGURE 13-1. Detailed Progression of How Research and Clinical Practice Are Integrated.

Source: Reprinted from Journal of the American Dietetic Association 98, Number 4 (April 1998), Eck, L.H., D.O. Slawson, R. Williams, K. Smith, K. Harmon-Clayton, and D. Oliver. "A Model for Making Outcomes Research Standard Practice in Clinical Dietetics," 455, Copyright 1998, with permission from Elsevier.

Table 13-1. Research Priorities

Core Research

A. Social Science Research

   1. Nutrition care that results in disease prevention/risk reduction or improves disease management throughout the life cycle
   2. Implementation and effectiveness of research findings for specific groups
   3. Behavioral change strategies for population groups and in settings
   4. Communication strategies to reach underserved groups
   5. New and innovation technologies for behavior change

B. Food Research

   1. Safe, secure, and sustainable food supply
   2. Expanded and updated food composition databases
   3. Safe food production and handling
   4. Food assistance programs in meeting population needs
   5. Individual choices on environment and food distribution system and people
   6. Nutritional value of changes in food composition availability

C. Basic Science and Nutrition Research

   1. Metabolic responses to modifications in intakes of bioactive food components
   2. Gene and genotype combinations likely to benefit from dietary modification
   3. Translating genomics and epigenetics research into the practice of dietetics

Dietetics Specific Research

A. Nutrition Care Process and Health Outcome Measures

   1. Accuracy and cost-effectiveness for assessing nutritional status
   2. Reliable and valid nutrition biomarkers of health outcomes
   3. Validity and usefulness of nutrition diagnoses to improve nutrition care outcomes

B. Delivery and Reimbursement of Dietetic Services

   1. Cost effectiveness of systems and technology for quality products and services
   2. Health outcome measures
   3. Effect of changes in the workforce on food and nutrition delivery
   4. Strategies for access to reimbursement for dietetic services
   5. Indicators for quality products and services in carious dietetic practice settings
   6. Cost-effective standards, measurements, tools in practice
   7. Customer satisfaction models and perceptions of value
   8. Drivers, barriers, and models for effectiveness of research findings in dietetic services

C. Dietetics Education and Retention

   1. Educational methods and strategies leading to competent practice
   2. Career paths for leadership positions
   3. Trends in employment of RDs and DTRs
   4. Attract and retain credentialed RDs and DTRs

RD = registered dietitian; DTR = dietetic technician, registered.
Source: Adapted from "Priorities for Research." Accessed June 20, 2012, www.eatright.org

Research Dietetic Practice Group

The Research Dietetic practice group has over 650 members from a variety of work settings, including clinical research centers, nonprofit groups, governmental agencies, universities, and many practice areas. Membership is open to all academy members who conduct research or are interested in research. Members collaborate on academy projects, such as the Evidence Analysis Library, to bring together research from many sources, and in the preparation of position papers. The academy estimates there are about 400 active researchers among the membership, and it would like to see this number increased.[8]

Members of this group also form liaisons with the Research Committee of the Association and the DPBRN. The practice group provides a member network, conducts continuing professional education events, provides a packet of information for new members, and produces a website and a periodic publication. Research awards are given to recognize the research and publications generated by members.

RESEARCH APPLICATIONS

Evidence-Based Practice

Evidence-based practice, based on evidence-based research, is the integration of the best available evidence from reviewed research with professional expertise and client values to make food and nutrition practice decisions.[9] Every area of practice in dietetics involves making decisions about the best procedures to follow, and given that new information continually leads to a need to make necessary changes or to update practice, evidence analysis provides this information. The evidence analysis process involves the following steps:

1. Formulate one or more questions to be researched.
2. Conduct a literature search for each question.
3. Critically appraise each report found in the literature as to the quality of the research and the findings.
4. Summarize the evidence.
5. Develop conclusions and assign a grade based on the strength of the evidence.
6. Put into practice.

The Evidence Analysis Library at the academy headquarters is maintained for the benefit of members of the academy and others needing the information. The best and most relevant nutrition information is reviewed and is available in an accessible, user-friendly library.[10] Because of the research data held, governmental and other groups also use the information and the process in making policy decisions. One example group is the Food and Drug Administration, which uses the process to make decisions about the use of health claims on food labels.

Outcomes research is increasingly important in the linkage of practice and research in order to make advancements in all areas of dietetics. Currently, translational research is being used in much the same way as outcomes research, that is, to link research to practice applications in all areas. Van Horn, editor-in chief of the *Journal of the Academy of Nutrition and Dietetics*, points out the value of clinical nutrition outcomes research and the involvement of dietitians in a letter in the journal.[11] Surveys show that while dietitians consider research important and are interested in it, many experience obstacles to performing outcomes research because of a lack of knowledge about the process, along with limited time and funding.[12,13] Dietetic educators and university faculty have also experienced barriers to research activities even though research is required of faculty.[14] The academy recently published an article linking job satisfaction of dietitians in management with research activities.[15]

INVOLVEMENT IN RESEARCH

The Commission on Dietetic Registration conducts periodic audits of practice areas of RDs and DTRs. In the most recent audit in 2010, data was collected for entry-level practitioners and is shown in **Table 13-2**. While the 2011 Compensation and Benefits Survey indicated that only 7 percent of RDs and 2 percent of DTRs are employed in education and research, the higher involvement in specific research-related activities in the practice audit would be expected to represent activities performed as a part of the job but not as the major area of employment.[16] The fact that dietetic technicians also participate in some research activities very likely reflects degrees obtained beyond the basic technician education requirements as well as job responsibilities.

Table 13-2. Research Activities of RDs and DTRs

	Percent Involved in Any Way	
	RD	**DTR**
Evaluate and synthesize research literature	19	10
Use evidence analysis in practice decisions	76	32
Review research literature	54	21
Evaluate and synthesize research literature	19	10
Use evidence analysis in practice decisions	76	32
Review research literature	54	21
Collect data for research	24	0
Analyze data	42	0
Write grant proposals	36	0
Develop hypotheses for research studies	5	0
Design research studies	6	0
Develop research proposals	5	0
Conduct research studies	8	0
Report research at professional conferences	6	0
Write manuscripts for peer-reviewed journals	5	0
Review and use national nutrition survey data	29	0
Identify nutrition-related problems within population groups.	12	0
Collect data for research	24	0
Analyze data	42	0
Write grant proposals	36	0
Develop hypotheses for research studies	5	0
Design research studies	6	0
Develop research proposals	5	0
Conduct research studies	8	0

Source: Reprinted from Journal of the American Dietetic Association 111, Number 11 (November 2011), Ward, B., D. Rogers, C. Mueller, R. Touger-Decker, KI.L. Sauer, C. Schmidt, "Distinguishing Entry-Level RD and DTR Practice: Results from the 2010 Commission on Dietetic Registration Entry-Level Dietetics Practice Audit, 1749–1755, Copyright 2011, with permission from Elsevier.

CAREER OPPORTUNITIES IN RESEARCH

Many university-affiliated hospitals have centers dedicated to types of clinical research. Others have long-term, multidisciplinary research projects that include a nutrition component. Some dietitians work at a general clinical research center (GCRC), usually associated with an academic medical center and federally funded. There are about 80 GCRCs funded by the National Institutes of Health located at universities across the country.

Research dietitians may oversee the metabolic kitchens associated with the GCRCs, analyze nutrient intakes, conduct calorimetry studies, assist in the development of nutrition-related protocols, and participate in rounds and seminars.

Some GCRC dietitians manage their own research programs, direct nutrition research, and collaborate with the medical school faculty in research. Some large national studies provide numerous opportunities for dietitians to become involved as nutrition counselors, data managers, or project directors.

Thee is a need for dietitians in clinical research. The best dietetics practice must be based on scientific principles and sound theory. Recent activities of the National Institutes of Health support these concepts.[17] In an attempt to advance the translation research activities into new drugs, equipment, new therapies for diseases, and prevention, it has established the National Center for Advancing Translational Science (NCATS). This center will fund projects and translational science centers all over the nation, which will provide dietitians and nutrition scientists with opportunities to collaborate with other scientists and compete for grants in applied research as basic science. Additional evidence is needed to support the value of many approaches to clinical dietetics. Additional knowledge is needed in areas of nutritional status of individuals and populations at risk for disease, genetic components of disease related to food intake patterns, identification of nutrient requirements associated with disease conditions, environmental risks (including dietary risks), nutrition interventions as therapy for disease conditions, and eating behavioral research. With the crises in healthcare delivery, especially in adult and childhood obesity, the outcomes of nutrition intervention are an important area of investigation.

Food and Industry Companies

Many food companies employ dietitians. Roles vary but include research related to product or recipe development. Roles can also focus on translation of research into meaningful information for the public or development of nutrition education for children, adults, and professionals.

Companies that manufacture infant formulas and medical nutritional products often employ dietitians to conduct research or to monitor clinical investigations in hospitals, nursing homes, and home care settings. Roles might include work related to:

- Nutritional needs of infants, children, and the elderly
- Acceptability of flavors and textures of products designed for oral use
- Coordination of studies to determine the effectiveness of new products
- Initiation of outcomes research to explore the cost-effectiveness of medical nutrition therapy

Government

There are many opportunities for research dietitians in government-sponsored centers and laboratories. These include positions such as:

- Nutrition scientists at the Department of Agriculture laboratories studying nutrient requirements, vitamins and minerals, eating pattern interventions, and other nutrition topics
- Researchers at the U.S. Army Natick Research, Development, and Engineering Center in Massachusetts involved in studies related to food behaviors and the acceptance and consumption of military rations
- Nutrition epidemiologists at the Centers for Disease Control and Prevention in Atlanta, Georgia, exploring patterns of nutrition-related-diseases and nutrition surveillance throughout the country
- Life science specialists at the Congressional Research Service in the Library of Congress, answering questions and conducting research for members of Congress and staff on food and nutrition issues
- Nutrition researchers at the National Aeronautical and Space Administration in Houston studying nutrition needs of space explorers

Community and Public Health

Since the leading causes of death in the United States continue to be nutrition-related chronic diseases, more efforts and opportunities are rising in community and population-based nutrition research. As consumers become more aware of disease consequences of their food choices and eating behaviors, they demand more evidence. Many dietitians who previously worked only in service program areas in community and public health are seizing the opportunity for research activities that document the value of nutrition and the dietitians' role in interventions. Great opportunities exist in conjunction with the obesity epidemic in getting individuals and communities involved in the food environment and in interventions that really change eating behaviors and adherence to dietary recommendations.

Schools are involved in research especially suited for nutrition, healthy behaviors, and weight maintenance by providing researchers access to students that they can follow over time. Dietitians will be needed in greater numbers for these research and education programs to be successful.

Many land-grant universities are conducting nutrition research in developing countries around the world. This research involves food and agriculture production, economic development, and nutritional assessment and intervention in various populations. As more and more globalization occurs, these ventures will increase, thus providing even greater opportunities for dietitians in research.

Human Nutrition Research Centers

The Agricultural Research Service of the U.S. Department of Agriculture funds six human nutrition research centers. These include the Children's Nutrition Research Center at Baylor College of Medicine in Houston, Texas, and the Arkansas Children's Nutrition Center at Arkansas Children's Hospital at the University of Arkansas for Medical Sciences. The center in Boston, Massachusetts, specializes in nutrition research for the aging population and is associated with Tufts University. Located on the campus of the University of California at Davis, the Western Human Nutrition Research Center concentrates on nutrition intervention strategies. The center in Beltsville, Maryland, conducts basic and applied research on nutrient composition, national dietary surveys, nutrient requirements, function of physiochemicals, and similar studies. The sixth center, located in Grand Forks, North Dakota, is associated with the

University of North Dakota and conducts research in mineral requirements and utilization as well as community-based research with Native Americans. Opportunities are available at these centers for all levels of dietetic practice (entry level, advanced, specialists, and dietetic technicians) and include clinical trials, basic science and applied research, and community-based research.

INFORMATION SOURCES

An excellent source for information about types of research and research methodology with an emphasis in nutrition is *Research: Successful Approaches* by Monsen and Van Horn.[18] The *Journal of the Academy of Nutrition and Dietetics* provides valuable research articles and opportunities identifying other dietetic researchers along with opportunities to publish. Other useful sources for dietitians conducting or planning research feature qualitative research,[19] publishing research,[20–22] and scientific integrity.[23,24] The Research Dietetics practice group offers opportunities for collaboration, networking, and mentoring for various kinds of research.

SUMMARY

Researchers may be based in specialized clinical research centers, government agencies, industry, universities, or the workplace. Roles vary according to the employing institution's mission and purpose. Key areas of investigation relate to nutrient requirements, nutrient utilization, and outcomes of medical nutrition therapy. Opportunities for participating in outcomes research in order to enhance practice exist through collaborative research that utilizes the expertise of dietitians in many practice settings. All dietitians can benefit from research findings applied to practice and can utilize the academy's Evidence Analysis Library for the current and best research.

DEFINITIONS

Evidence-based research. The compilation of research studies that, together, allow for a decision regarding application to practice.
Outcomes research. Studies that focus on results of interventions and application of research results.

Research. Systematic investigation leading to new knowledge or new applications of known information. To conduct research, a question is formulated, a literature search is conducted, experimental activities are applied, and results are recorded.

REFERENCES

1. Pavlinac, J.M. "President's Page." *J Am Diet Assoc* 110 (2010): 499.
2. Trostler, N., E.F. Meyer, and L.G. Snetselaar. "Description of Practice Characteristics and Professional Activities of Dietetics Practice-Based Research Network Members." *J Am Diet Assoc* 108 (2008): 1060–1067.
3. Yadrick, M. "President's Page." *J Am Diet Assoc* 109 (2008): 11601.
4. See Note 1.
5. "Priorities for Research." Academy of Dietetics and Nutrition, Accessed March 10, 2012, www.eatright.org
6. Academy of Nutrition and Dietetics. "Research: Philosophy and Framework." Accessed December 19, 2012, www.eatright.org
7. See Note 1.
8. See Note 5.
9. Vaughn, L.A., and C.J.J. Manning. "Meeting the Challenges of Dietetics Practice with Evidence-Based Decisions." *J Am Diet Assoc* 104 (2004): 282–284.
10. Academy of Dietetics and Nutrition. "Evidence-Based Library," Accessed April 1, 2012, www.eatright.org
11. Van Horn, L. "Clinical Nutrition Research: New Approaches and New Outcomes." *Acad Nutr Diet J* 112 (2012): 971.
12. McCaffree, J. "Overcoming Obstacles to Outcomes Research." *J Am Diet Assoc* 102 (2002): 71.
13. Hayes, J.E., and C.A. Peterson. "Use of an Outcomes Research Collaborative Training Curriculum to Enhance Entry-Level Dietitians and Established Professionals' Self-Reported Understanding of Research." *J Am Diet Assoc* 103 (2003): 77–81.
14. Whelan, K., and S. Markless. "Factors That Influence Research Involvement among Registered Dietitians Working as University Faculty: A Qualitative Interview Study." *Acad Nutr Diet J* 112 (2012): 1021–1028.
15. Sauer, K., D. Canter, and C. Shanklin. "Job Satisfaction of Dietitians with Management Responsibilities: An Exploratory Study Supporting ADAs Research Priorities." *Acad Nutr Diet J* 112, Suppl. (2012): S6–S11.
16. Ward, B., D. Rogers, C. Mueller, R. Touger-Decker, K. Sauer, and D. Schmidt. "Distinguishing Entry-Level RD and DTR Practice: Results from the 2010 Commission on Dietetic Registration Entry-Level Dietetics Practice Audit." *J Am Diet Assoc* 111 (2011): 1749–1755.
17. U.S. Department of Health and Human Services. "NIH Establishes National Center for Advancing Translational Sciences." *NIH News*, press release, December 23, 2011.

18 Monson, E.R., and L. Van Horn. *Research, Successful Approaches*, 3rd ed. (Chicago: American Dietetic Association, 2007).

19. Harris, J.E., G.P.M. Gleason, C.Boushey, J.A. Beto, and B. Bruemer. "An Introduction to Qualitative Research for Food and Nutrition Professionals." *J Am Diet Assoc* 109 (2009): 80–90.

20. Boushey, C., J. Harris, B. Bruemmer, S. L. Archer, and L. Van Horn. "Publishing Nutrition Research: A Review of Study Design, Statistical Analyses, and Other Key Elements of Manuscript Preparation. Part 1." *J Am Diet Assoc* 106 (2006): 89–96.

21. Harris, J.E., C. Boushey, B. Bruemmer, and S.A. Archer. "Publishing Nutrition Research: A Review of Nonparametric Methods." *J Am Diet Assoc* 108 (2008): 1488–1496.

22. Boushey, C.J., J. Harris, B. Bruemmer, and S.L. Archer. "Publishing Nutrition Research: A Review of Sampling, Sample Size, Statistical Analyses, and Other Key Elements of Manuscript Preparation. Part 2." *J Am Diet Assoc* 108 (2008): 679–688.

23. The International Life Sciences Institute North America Conflict of Interest/ Scientific Integrity Guiding Principles Working Group. "Funding Food Science and Nutrition Research: Financial Conflicts and Scientific Integrity." *J Am Diet Assoc* 109 (2009): 929–936.

24. Nicklas, T.S., W. Karmally, and C.E. O'Neil. "Nutrition Professionals Are Obligated to Follow Ethical Guidelines When Conducting Industry-Funded Research." *J Am Diet Assoc* 111 (2011): 1931–1932.

CHAPTER 14

The Future in Dietetics

"The Dogma of the quiet past are inadequate for the stormy present and future. As our circumstances are new, we must think anew, and act anew."
Abraham Lincoln

INTRODUCTION

The dietetics profession is facing unprecedented challenges and changes that will impact practice in many ways. The economic climate of doing more with less is expected to continue and have implications for the present outlook and continued employment for dietitians. Traditional institutions, such as hospitals, schools, public health agencies, businesses, and universities, all face restructuring and downsizing of workforces at the same time there is increased interest in nutrition, food, health, and wellness. Even more diverse populations are expected to increase in the future, giving urgency to professionals prepared to work with many different groups and across ethnic and cultural differences.

Significant trends that will reshape the profession are changing demographics, globalization, increasing consumer expectations, the technological revolution, and health care. In a rapidly changing environment, a proactive understanding of the changing healthcare market, development of new global competencies and capabilities, and a shift from tangible assets to an appreciation of the value of knowledge and technology will be needed. As a helping profession founded to promote the welfare of all citizens, the Academy of Nutrition and Dietetics is poised to help meet the challenges presented by the many forces impacting the lives of individuals and communities.

CHANGING DEMOGRAPHICS

The U.S. Census Bureau estimates the U.S. population will be about 430 million by 2050.[1] It is further estimated that 50 percent of the population will be white non-Hispanic, 14 percent black, 24 percent Hispanic, 8 percent Asian, and 4 percent other. The age distribution is rapidly undergoing changes as well—a shift from a higher percentage of the young to those over age 65. White males born in 2006 have a life expectancy of 76 years, but black males have a life expectancy of 70 years. White females can expect to live 81 years compared with 77 years for black females.[2] The incidence of chronic disease will likely increase and will greatly affect healthcare and healthcare costs. The mobility of the population, women working away from home, and the gap between "haves" and "have-nots" leading to food insecurity and dependence on government support all have implications for the kind and amount of nutrition support needed from dietitians.

Ethnic Diversity

Ethnic foods, cultural practices, and language all present challenges for health professionals working with persons with different ethnic backgrounds. Knowledge about nutritional values of ethnic foods, understanding of cultural views on health and nutrition in general, and ways of communicating and counseling will be increasingly important for the profession.

As the fastest growing population group, Latinos, compared with whites, experience significantly higher rates of poverty, food insecurity, depression, lack of leisure time and related physical activity, obesity, and diabetes.[3] A study of acculturation and diet among Latinos, principally in California, concluded that the less acculturated may need more emphasis on dietary choices and food preparation practices while the more acculturated may benefit from messages that emphasize moderation in the use of fast food, sugar-sweetened beverages, and other away-from-home foods.[4]

The *Code of Ethics for the Profession of Dietetics* addresses the issue of meeting the needs of diverse populations.[5] Principle 3 states, "the dietetics practitioner considers the health, safety, and welfare of the public at all times"[6] and Principle 5 says, "the dietetics practitioner provides professional services with objectivity and respect for the unique needs and values of individuals."[7]

Racial and ethnic health disparities affect minority populations disproportionately but affect everyone. Food and nutrition professionals play a key role in reducing these health differences. The most effective care is equitable, respectful, and compatible with the language, culture, and health beliefs of those they serve.[8]

Age Diversity

Baby boomers are driving many of the health and nutrition practices today; however, both older and younger generations have ingrained attitudes that differ in some dramatic ways (**Table 14-1**). Fast-food preferences, image perceptions, and a tendency to turn to supplements for their nutrition concerns are among some of the characteristics of generations that followed the baby boomers. The newer generation Z, or those born between 1994 and 2004, are also known as the Internet generation, and they are used to multitasking and using many technological tools.[9] Reaching them with health messages will be increasingly by distance and online.

Table 14-1. Generational Attitudes and Values Toward Food and Nutrition

Attitude/Value	Silent Generation (born before 1945)	Baby Boomers (born 1946–1964)	Generation X (born 1965–1985)	Gen Y (born 1986–present)
Attitudes to nutrition, health	Those aged 60–70 not silent and seeking more variety and more healthful choices. Have health concerns and interested in better diets.	A bit more active and exercise more. Trying to eat healthfully, more interested in nutrition, longevity.	More fast foods. Like supplements for health maintenance. May be uneducated about nutrition, but older Xers are getting the diet–health connection.	Want to know where the food comes from, how it was produced. Interested in organics.
Attitudes to nutrition, health	Don't want to waste food. Will exercise. Attribute health to moderate diet, daily activity, and not smoking.	Want to spend the second half of life healthy but over-ambitious in making changes.	Permissive parents, allow children to decide what to eat—kids can nag for favorite foods. Alternatively, pressure kids to be perfect.	Use supplements for the quick fix. The generation of artificial food stuffs, fast foods, with some exercise.
Attitudes to nutrition, health	Still have gardens, shop frugally, and know how to prepare, store food.	Have food skills, but financial freedom not to use. Some attracted to alternative medicines, others drug-reliant for health, mood.	Producing a generation of overweight children—high-energy snacks, little exercise. Interested in diet only when pregnant or caring for infants.	
Fads and new food habits	Eating out—we've earned it!	Acquired Starbucks habit, reverting to cocktails later in the day. Eating out or takeout because busy. Boomers always extremists.	Starbucks trendy drinks are the new cocktails for this generation. This is the fad diet generation. Sipping from water bottles all day. Confusion about carbohydrates and vegetarianism.	Sipping from water bottles all day. Restaurants are models for meals. Prefer eating out. Would prefer to drink their meals (e.g., supplements, fortified waters). Confusion about carbohydrates and vegetarianism.

Obsession with body image	Not a big concern.	High value: Self-absorbed and self-rationalizing: eating disorders kept secret, even from doctors and families.	High value: More open about eating disorders. Health less important than image.	High value: More open about eating disorders.
Changes in family life	Some experience with changes. Becoming more like Boomers in their family life.	Family meals rare and precious. Lack of time means quick food prep.	Many variations in family makeup, more single households. May not cook.	Norm: Everyone in the family operates individually. Can't cook, do not want to.
Approaches to life/work	Live to work, or did before they retired. Have had to learn the most: technologies, culture change, and so on.	Motivated by status, power, need for money to fund luxury lifestyles, work all hours.	Motivated by status, power, need for money to fund luxury lifestyles, work all hours. Less loyalty to employers, more turnover.	Less loyalty and desire to please employers. Expect autonomy and self-direction, high-status jobs, but overall, less driven.
Health: chronic problems	Need a diagnosis before acting.	More motivated to take charge of chronic conditions. Maybe half face heart attacks, diabetes, obesity.	More motivated to take charge of chronic conditions, and make changes before problems occur.	Want more information about chronic disease, learning about diabetes at a young age.
Educational strategies, concerns	Range from "too late to change now," to those with free time and interest in new strategies. Respectful and willing to listen.	Information NOW demanded. May be in denial and avoid learning. Older Boomers more willing to listen.	Willing to help with "causes" and be involved. Unsure of how to implement change. Information NOW demanded. Can be confrontational. Will pick and choose to suit what they want.	Needs entertainment to get the message. Wants information personalized—no groups! Information NOW demanded.

(continues)

Table 14-1. Generational Attitudes and Values Toward Food and Nutrition *(continued)*

Attitude/Value	Silent Generation (born before 1945)	Baby Boomers (born 1946–1964)	Generation X (born 1965–1985)	Gen Y (born 1986–present)
Dealing with growing older, diet, living, change, attitudes to the future	May be the last meat and potatoes generation. Will be slow, steady in change. Do what the doctor says, even when no longer relevant. Entitlement attitude may overwhelm social services/ health care.	Still want center stage, won't be run off. Will want more ethnic influence and variety in assisted-living dining. More stress, seeking balance in busy lives, but question everything. "Live for the day" attitude, no concern for future health.	More questioning of the status quo and of authority. Want to negotiate change, prefer a quick fix, the magic pill, not to do the work. Are hardworking on their own terms, not including working on their own health, cooking meals, too busy. "Live for the day" attitude, no concern for future health. May become more concerned for their children's habits, health.	Invincibility of youth, unaware of long-term effects. Have heard the nutrition message in school—effect yet to be seen. Food an opportunity for casual contact, not long-term relationships. "It's not my problem" attitude. "Live for the day" attitude, no concern for future health.

Source: Reprinted from Journal of the American Dietetic Association 107, Number 7 (July 2007), Jarrat, J., and J.B. Mahaffle. "The Profession of Dietetics at a Critical Juncture: A Report on the 2006 Environmental Scan for the American Dietetic Association," S39–S57, Copyright 2007, with permission from Elsevier.

Their reliance on technology means more time is spent indoors and in a sedentary life, leading to health consequences. Their ability to work in teams and in collaborative ways will need to be considered by employers in the future. Both educators and employers will need to be aware of this age group's strengths in the use of technology and also the implications of their lifestyle and how they have learned.

Aging Population

The life expectancy in the United States has increased over the years due in great part to better medical screening and treatment along with advances in treatments for some chronic diseases.[10] While cardiovascular disease and cancer death rates have dropped, others such as Alzheimer's disease, kidney disease, hypertension, and Parkinson's disease have increased. Further, obesity-related conditions are poised to increase in the future.[11]

The oldest old—those aged 85 and older—have become the fastest growing group among all age groups. The population of this group is expected to grow by 377 percent by the year 2050.[12] This group is also at higher risk for many preventable health problems; almost 75 percent have at least one chronic illness. There is also a rise in disability among those aged 50 to 64, years leading to high unemployment and the need for more home care.[13] The unfortunate reality of modern health care is that it is focused more on treatment than prevention of chronic disease. This area of practice presents dietitians great opportunities for preventing chronic disease and disability in older patients by counseling in health and wellness programs, in outpatient clinics, home care, and nutrition services in retirement and assisted living centers. Sayhoun recommends specific steps dietitians can take to be proactive in providing services to the aging population.[14]

HEALTH AND WELLNESS

Because healthcare costs have a tremendous influence on the country's economy, the whole healthcare system is being reshaped. With the 2010 Patient Protection and Affordable Care Act (HR 3590), many reforms in the current healthcare system are expected to expand healthcare coverage and reduce healthcare costs. As the reforms occur, the healthcare system will be reoriented away from acute disease management toward preventive care and wellness, and healthcare services will be more inte-grated.[15] One concept with potential for dietitians is the patient-centered medical home, which coordinates care for both children and adults with primary care physicians (i.e., pediatricians and family practice, etc.), coor-dinating care on a continuum which emphasizes prevention and chronic care. Dietitians can be an essential member of the team as nutrition care is so much a part of prevention of the most prevalent chronic diseases (e.g., obesity, hypertension, and diabetes).

Further changes in the healthcare system are likely to occur in the next decade due to Medicare and Medicaid changes in reimbursements for medical care. While medical nutrition therapy has been very effective in providing nutritional care and reimbursement to dietitians who practice in particular clinical areas, efforts to expand the coverage to other disease conditions have not been successful. This is an issue in public policy in which dietitians can play an important part.

Health and wellness is poised to receive increasing attention as the obe-sity epidemic expands with serious effects on public resources as well as health. The early development of chronic diseases and shortened life spans are of great concern to the medical profession and researchers. The Healthy People 2020 initiative by the National Institutes of Health reflects a vision of a society in which all people live long, healthy lives.[16] Many factors—societal, economic, and political—will help determine the success of this ambitious goal for the U.S. population. Dietitians are on the forefront of helping make this happen by the services they are prepared to provide.

The academy foundation has named childhood obesity as a high priority area for both educational and funding efforts. Schools have an important role to play in overcoming the growing incidence of childhood obesity through the school food service programs and nutrition education.

The relationship between risk factors, health outcomes, and nutrition is shown in **Figure 14-1**.

COMMUNICATIONS

In a recent practice paper of the academy, the following description of communication today summed up the situation: "today's informa-tion landscape—a whole new world."[17] The means of communication today have greatly increased and will continue to evolve in the future. Media sources of information include television, radio, newspapers,

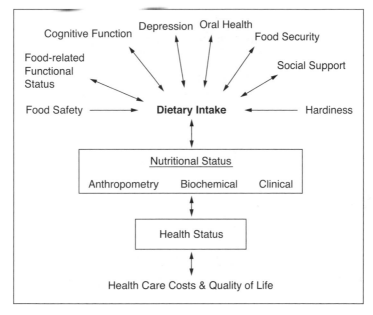

FIGURE 14-1. Relationship Between Risk Factors, Health Outcomes, and Nutrition.

Source: Reprinted from Journal of the American Dietetic Association 111, no. 6 (June 2011), Nadine R. Sahyoun, "Expanding Opportunities for Registered Dietitians in the Health Care System," 813–815, Copyright 2011, with permission from Elsevier.

and magazines as well as websites, blogs, videos, social networking services, phone applications, and even advertising and food packaging.

The many ways of providing information hold both benefits and challenges for dietetics professionals as well as consumers. This is evidenced in the way other individuals, the food industry, other health professionals, personal trainers, health food store employees, as well as self-styled experts freely give food and nutrition advice to the public. **Figure 14-2** shows the sources of nutrition information for the public. It is evident that registered dietitians (RDs) have many competitors and are actually far down the list of the most influential providers.

The line between misinformation and accurate, science-based food and nutrition information is also difficult to discern, especially given the many sources. This presents another very important area of need the RD can fulfill in working with clients, patients, and groups.[18,19]

A 2011 survey conducted by the American Dietetic Association (ADA) Nutrition Informatics Committee showed the extent to which dietitians used technology and information management.[20] Among those surveyed,

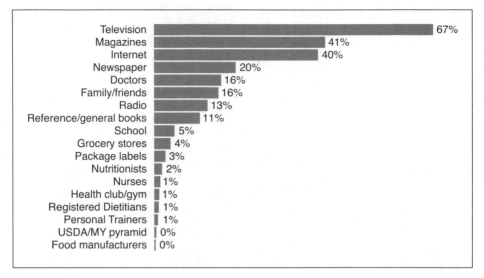

FIGURE 14-2. Sources of Nutrition Information for the Public.

Source: Reproduced from: Position Paper of the Academy of Nutrition and Dietetics, "Communicating about Food and Nutrition Information," 2012, www.eatright.org, drawn from the "Nutrition and You: Trends 2011" national public opinion survey conducted by the Academy of Nutrition and Dietetics (then known as the American Dietetic Association). Accessed August 20, 2012.

62 percent indicated they were experienced or highly experienced in using and retaining electronic data. Fifty-two percent strongly agreed that they use data and technology to problem solve.[21]

The academy is rapidly turning to electronic means to transmit a great deal of information to professionals and to consumers. These include the following:

For Professionals
- *Electronic journal*: *Journal of the Academy of Nutrition and Dietetics* and archives of past issues.
- *Electronic magazine*: *Food and Nutrition* magazine.
- *Electronic newsletters*: *Behind the Scenes at the Academy*, ACEND newsletter online, *Eat Right Weekly*, *MNT Provider*, and *Student Scoop*.
- *E-mail*: Updates daily.
- *Advertising*

For Consumers
- EatRight Radio—public service announcements
- National Media Spokespersons program
- Website at www.eatright.org

INFORMATION TECHNOLOGY AND MANAGEMENT

Information and communication technologies are a fact of life in both work and personal lives. Individuals engage with technology in order to get work accomplished; this is increasingly true in all areas of dietetics. Using technology to stay in touch with clients may improve eating and exercise compliance and create new business opportunities. Clients can use their phones to take photos of meals and interact with a dietitian using an interactive software tool called MealLogger.[22] The service is being used in hospitals, universities, by corporate wellness service providers, fitness clubs and individual dietitians. Another example of technology use with implications in food service organizations is service-oriented architecture (SOA) software to design systems that computerize many business activities.[23]

Recent research points to an area of technology use termed *technostress* that affects users directly.[24] By looking at several characteristics of technology, it is hypothesized that work overload and role ambiguity are the main stressors. Such stress effects may impact productivity and the quality of work life in the work environment. Technostress is an area of research that will likely receive more attention in the future as it affects RDs and dietetic technicians, registered (DTRs).

ENVIRONMENTAL ISSUES

The trend toward living green is one that will continue to grow as more consumers turn to organic, locally grown foods and ecofriendly, household supplies. Organic foods and beverages are fast-growing segments of the large food market today.[25] Reducing waste by recycling leads to significant reductions in environmental pollutants as well as overflowing landfills. Schools, health care, and commercial operations generate 35 to 45 percent of the total municipal solid waste in the United States, giving rise to the need for awareness and steps to handle waste items in more ecofriendly ways.[26]

Other issues in environmental sustainability are energy and water consumption. Dietitians and those in commercial food establishments need to help select energy-saving equipment and take steps to reduce the amount of water and energy used in food production. Examples of going green in hospitals, such as using flexible menus in order to make the best use of foods in season, buying from local farmers and producers, and checking all processes for the best energy and water usage were discussed in an issue of the *ADA Times*.[27] The sustainability of the food supply, as well as the nutritional quality of foods, especially those that must be transported long distances over significant periods of time, must also be taken into consideration by dietitians. The cost of energy for the travel and costs of food that may have to be discarded must be figured into the greening of food systems.

Even greener meetings need to be a goal of all professionals. This means meetings that minimize water and energy use, from the distance traveled to the meeting to the type and amount of food and water used, the energy used in lighting and electricity, the paper and plastic recycled, and the amount of waste left behind.[28]

NUTRIGENOMICS

Genetic dietetics is a term becoming increasingly familiar as researchers publish findings about genetics and its role in health care. DeBusk and others are alerting dietitians to the potential for individualized treatments and diets designed for each person's genetic makeup.[29-31] A whole new field is evolving based on nutrigenomics, or the scientific study of the way specific genes and bioactive food components interact.[32] Dietitians will be key in the development of this concept and this research as they represent the discipline with the greatest knowledge in nutrient composition of foods and the metabolism of food and have taken leadership roles in developing and improving dietary assessment methodology, all critical to the genomic research.[33,34]

Genetic knowledge may eventually be used in the future to avert childhood and adult obesity, metabolic syndromes, heart disease, and many other nutrition-related disorders. Nutrigenomics information may well be a part of dietetics practice in the future, and standards of practice in regard to disclosure and privacy will be needed in working with patients and clients.[35]

Other "omics" are also being identified, namely, proteomics and metabolomics (**Figure 14-3**). Another term, *epigenetics*, is described as the way that environmental factors, such as food and supplement intake, can

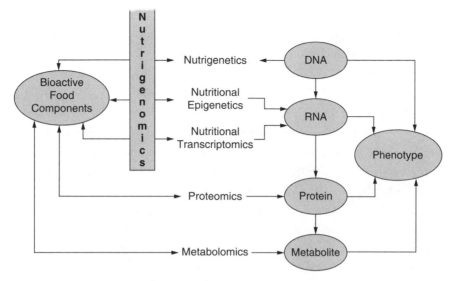

FIGURE 14-3. Nutritional "Omics."

Source: Reprinted from Journal of the American Dietetic Association 106, Number 3 (March 2006), Trujllo, E., C. Davis, and J. Milner. "Nutrigenomics, Proteomics, Metabolomics, and the Practice of Dietetics," 403–413, Copyright 2006, with permission from Elsevier.

alter gene activity and thereby affect cellular function and metabolism.[36] Dietitians will be at the forefront collaborating with genetic scientists in evaluating, translating, and applying this research for individual clients/ patients and for the public in general. Dietetic practitioners with specialty training will be needed to conduct health assessments and counsel patients when these procedures are used. Expansion of food composition data, innovative dietary assessment methods, new diagnostic tests, changes in the dietary reference intakes (DRIs), and specialty foods are projected to occur in dietetics to support this new area.[37,38]

Nanotechnology and nanoscale science are rapidly changing the environment of food production, food safety and quality, and food packaging, causing the Food and Drug Administration to establish the Nanotechnology Task Force to determine the regulatory challenges and need for new regulations.[39] The potential is great and offers exciting new possibilities in applications in nutritional science and dietetics practice.[40,41] New nutrient delivery systems, improvements in food safety and sanitation practices, and increases in the number of enriched and fortified food products may be possible with this new technology.

These new areas of science and research have profound implications for the dietetics profession, including continuing education and collaboration with scientists as crucial needs now and in the near future. Positive attitudes are important, but knowledge is essential for incorporating the new processes and procedures into practice.[42]

COLLABORATION WITH OTHER PROFESSIONALS

Health care is the shared responsibility of medical and allied health professionals who are the most effective when information and work is shared. The academy maintains ties with many allied health professions realizing that an appreciation for what each can provide is vital to the success of all. In the modern hospital, many professions and many systems play roles, among which dietitians are one key part. In the community, many other institutions also provide care. Pharmacies, pharmaceutical companies, equipment manufacturers, home health and assistive devices providers all help fill critical needs. The nanoscience area discussed previously underscores the need for the dietitian of the future to communicate and collaborate with food technologists, food scientists, and food production and manufacturing agents, and to be knowledgeable of their scientific language through their publications.

An interesting study in Australia highlighted the role nurses play in helping provide nutritional care.[43] It was emphasized that there is a role for nurses in observing; participating in screening for development of care plans; giving support in feeding, both enteral and parenteral; and working with dietary staff to manage periods of noneating, changes in eating behavior, and changes in the physical condition of patients such as weight loss.

Nutritional pharmacology is a term applied to the many interactions between nutrition care and medicine.[44] Genetic differences affect the individual's reaction to both nutritional factors and medicines. Potential therapeutic roles have been documented for many vitamins, minerals, amino acids, fatty acids, and accessory nutrients such as coenzyme Q and phytochemicals. As the field of nutrigenomics advances, dietitians may assume a larger role in the even more effective use of nutrients in treatment and collaborate with pharmacists in making these decisions.

FUTURE ROLES IN DIETETICS

Opportunities in Health Care

The healthcare industry continues to grow, and the cost of medical care rises along with advances in care, new procedures that are developed, and the aging population. Several forces bolster the growth and the cost. They include[45]:

- Advances in medical technology
- Aging
- Insufficient preventive care
- Government healthcare oversight and mandates
- Medicalization of more conditions
- Malpractice legal actions

Because of these trends and rising health costs, emphasis on preventive medicine is growing. Following this trend, the National Institutes of Health issues its Healthy People goals each decade, targeting specific disease conditions and environmental, societal, and communication needs toward improving the overall health of Americans.

As healthcare reform takes shape and whether there is significant action now or in the future, there are a number of ways dietitians can help influence and be ready for reform. These include the following[46]:

- Participate in wellness and preventive initiatives
- Assume excellent patient satisfaction
- Embrace electronic health records
- Identify community partners and get involved in community needs assessment programs and efforts
- Prepare for growth in outpatient activity
- Network with peers
- Be prepared for e-visits

An interesting concept discussed in *The Futurist* suggests that the traditional hospital should shift to a "healthspital" with an emphasis on a holistic and more expansive view of health care that embraces wellness and prevention of disease.[47] Data and information management, use of remote monitoring, involvment of patients and families in information and support networks, and promotion of healthy lifestyles for all would be characteristics of such a shift.

The demand for dietetic professionals is expected to grow as fast as the average for all industries in the nation's economy. There will be a need for increased meals and nutrition programs in long-term care, schools, correctional institutions, residential care, community health, home health care, and health and fitness clubs, among others. Traditional professional roles (such as food service administrator or clinical practitioner) will almost become obsolete in the future. The new healthcare environment will see dietetic professionals managing multiple departments or providing transdisciplinary health services, in which nutrition is only part of the practice role. In the future, it will not be uncommon to see food and nutrition experts earn dual degrees, with the second degrees being in medicine, pharmacy, nursing, physical therapy, business, law, or hotel and restaurant management.

Additionally, there will be some executive-level positions in integrated health systems and in traditional healthcare organizations. These positions will require a new set of competencies in such areas as strategic planning, information management, marketing, finance, and cost-benefit analyses. An academy leader in advanced level practice, Linda Lafferty, indicates that this area will

> employ the concepts of production/operations management and quantitative business analysis. Decision-making individuals at these levels are fluent in the language already. This is a compelling reason for RDs in management (regardless of area of dietetic practice) to be able to speak this language.[48]

Advanced practice in dietetics of the future may require advanced degrees in areas like business (such as an MBA), systems management, etc. Supplement 1 of the March 2012, *Academy of Nutrition and Dietetics Journal* has a series of articles on workforce demands and recommendations for the future in dietetics.[49]

Food

Consumers want new foods and foods that are safe, healthful, and economical. Convenience will continue to drive demand, which accounts for the continuing popularity of fast foods and easily obtainable food. New demands will be made for healthy fast food and drive-through restaurants. Special food for segments of the population will also drive demand, especially the aging and those on weight-loss diets. The growing epidemic of obesity among children as well as adults means that dietitians with multiple backgrounds in food science, culinary arts, food product development, and exercise and fitness are and will continue to be in demand. Greater emphasis will be placed on community involvement in solving the problems of preventing obesity, which will increase the need for involvement of dietitians in intervention research, community health, and public health.

The commercial food service industry will continue to provide careers for those interested in combining an interest in foods, international cuisine, and business administration. Restaurants and in-home catering will grow as consumers entertain more, cook less, and eat away from home. Resorts hire food professionals. Food manufacturers and food distributors look to members of the profession who can provide marketing support, sales training, new product development, and food photography support. Many hotels are setting up educational child care centers for parents traveling with children; they need help with nutrition education programming, health and fitness programs, and developmentally appropriate feeding strategies. Associations representing health professions are also employing food and nutrition consultants to help develop transdisciplinary education programs.

The foods and food service industries will continue to gain public attention as restaurant menu labeling, the Dietary Guidelines for Americans, functional foods, and even increasing food costs are discussed in news media.[50,51] Governmental policies have tremendous impact on the overall food industry through the issuance of eating guides, regulations for school nutrition programs and senior nutrition programs, and congressional guidance in the farm bill (reissued every 5 years). All these areas also present greater potential employment areas for dietitians.

Research

With continually advancing information, new opportunities will exist for those interested in the discovery of knowledge through research. There is a need for those interested in studying both nutrition science and nutrition intervention issues and problems through continuing and advanced study. New and emerging clinical protocols, intervention trials, and cost-benefit studies must be tested. Genetics and biotechnology are driving the need for discovery as the effects on food and nutrition are being explored and the information is made available to consumers. Similarly, there is a need for food researchers who want to develop new products or who want to understand consumer satisfaction and service quality factors. Marketing research also has tremendous growth potential as advances in the food delivery system must be modeled, simulated, and tested for quality, efficiency, cost-effectiveness, and consumer acceptance.

Public Service

Public service and the military offer opportunities for the dietetics professional with many benefits and a range of activities. Military dietitians, for instance, fulfill a variety of roles today, from running healthcare facilities stateside and abroad, to filling teaching and research positions, to creating health and wellness programs. Over time, military RDs can move into management, such as hospital administration, one of the many opportunities for upward mobility.

Governmental agencies such as the U.S. Department of Agriculture and Health and Human Services, Congress, and governmental–industry associations such as the International Food Information Council employ dietitians. Others work in international food organizations such as the United Nations Food and Agriculture Organization (FAO). In these positions, they serve in policy development, consumer information, food and nutrition research, and school nutrition and food safety programs. Dietitians serve on the Dietary Guidelines for Americans and MyPlate planning groups. Others work for the food and nutrition board of the National Academy of Sciences developing various recommendations and standards regarding nutrition, and food, including the dietary reference intakes (DRIs).[52]

These positions and others in public service offer opportunities that require innovation, motivation, and a willingness to set out on what can be quite different paths. Dietitians will serve as lobbyists in the future and run for public office at every level of government.

PLANNING FOR THE FUTURE

In addressing the future, dietitians must meet the challenges brought about as a result of reengineering both the health delivery system and the food industry. Those individuals who can capitalize on future trends, who understand how basic assumptions will change dietetic practice and who proactively search out new career opportunities will be well poised for the future. Others who believe the future is more of the same will find their positions disappearing—even after many years of dedicated service.

The profession must always expect the unexpected and assume the future is not an extension of the past. There are several assumptions that can be made about the future that will guide dietetic professionals in making career decisions. These assumptions include:

- The ability to connect and communicate effectively electronically will continue to revolutionize how, when, and where dietetic professionals will practice.
- Professionals, not the organizations' management, will emerge as primary players in multidisciplinary teams; managers will become facilitators, coaches, and mentors.
- The concept of organization will expand to include links to all external partners, including consumers.
- Most people will be connected, worldwide, forming new professional opportunities and risks.
- Services and products that dietetic professionals offer to clients will be "informationalized"; databases will be built into more products, programs, and services offered to consumers.
- Competition will no longer be limited to local, regional, or national audiences; it will be worldwide.
- Continual and timely learning will be the rule for health providers and their clients.
- Most individuals will study and live within multicultural settings and among people speaking multiple languages.
- Professionals will become more entrepreneurial and innovative in their approach to career design.

As discussed, turbulent times create both opportunities and threats for members of the profession. How should individual members shape their careers to fit into future scenarios? Steps that can be taken are:

- Be visionary and manage your own career. Make a conscious shift of mind not to rely on traditional practice roles. Be open to future opportunities.
- Build a portfolio of education and skills that will position you for future career changes. There will be a need for people who can

increase productivity with limited resources and who can develop cost-effective solutions to problems.

- If you are not technologically literate, become so. Be able to design organizational and consumer programs that use multiple multimedia approaches and formats.
- Be adept at building relationships, both internal and external, to the profession. A distinct competitive advantage will come to those who know how to network, connect, and communicate with consumers, experts, and information specialists.
- Become an expert at accessing, acquiring, disseminating, and evaluating knowledge. It is the key strategic resource.
- Consider working at the periphery of the profession and related professions and seek out new areas.
- The most critical skills that will be needed for success in the future include computer skills, statistical analyses, communication skills, financial management, critical analysis, strategic planning, and negotiation. Success also calls for an entrepreneurial outlook and motivation.

SUMMARY

The dietetic profession is changing and becoming increasingly responsive to the needs of consumers and the marketplace. Because of changes in population demographics, increasing globalization, and changes in the healthcare system, the profession is faced with unprecedented challenges, but also great opportunities. Planning toward and preparing for the future through acquiring appropriate education and developing technical and personal skills such as acquisition and dissemination of knowledge, leadership qualities, and willingness to change will serve the dietitian well into the future.

DEFINITIONS

Allied health professions. Healthcare organizations or groups providing services that supplement and assist those in direct health care.

Demographics. Population statistics relating to characteristics of those making up the population, such as births, deaths, and ages that are used in various ways.

Epigenetics. Environmental factors that can alter gene activity and metabolism.

Genetic dietetics. The translation of the interaction of genes and environmental factors into clinical applications to improve nutritional health outcomes.

Multicultural. Different cultures found in populations.

Multidisciplinary. A collection of several disciplines either similar or diverse in nature.

REFERENCES

1. Haughton, B., and J. Stang. "Population Risk Factors and Trends in Health Care and Public Policy." *Acad Nutr Diet J* 112, Suppl. 1 (2012): S35–S46.
2. See Note 1.
3. Perez-Escamilla, R. "Dietary Quality Among Latinos: Is Acculturation Making Us Sick?" *J Am Diet Assoc* 106 (2006): 988–991.
4. Ayala, G.X., Baquery, B., and S. Klinger. "A Systematic Review of the Relationship between Acculturation and Diet Among Latinos in the United States: Implications for Future Research." *J Am Diet Assoc* 108 (2008): 1330–1334.
5. Fileti, C.P. "Ethics Opinion: Eliminating Dietetics-Related Inequalities." *J Am Diet Assoc* 111 (2011): 307–309.
6. "American Dietetic Association/Commission on Dietetic Registration Code of Ethics for the Profession of Dietetics and process for Consideration of Ethical Issues." *J Am Diet Assoc* 2009 (109): 1461–1465.
7. See Note 6.
8. Johnson-Askew, W.L., L. Gordon, and S. Sockalingam. "Practice Paper of the American Dietetic Association: Addressing Racial and Ethnic Health Disparities." *J Am Diet Assoc* 111 (20112): 446–456.
9. Wikipedia. "Generation Z." Accessed June 18, 2012, www.en.wikipedia.org/wiki/generation_Z
10. Centers for Disease Control and Prevention. "Life Expectancy." Accessed June 22, 2012, www.cdc.gov/nchs
11. HealthyPeople.gov. "Healthy People 2020." Accessed June 1, 2012, www.healthypeople.gov
12. Rhea, M., and C. Bettles. "Future Changes Driving Dietetics Workforce Supply and Demand: Future Scan 2012–2022." *Acad Nutr Diet J* 112 (2012): S10–S24.
13. See Note 12.
14. Sayhoun, N.R. "Expanding Opportunities for Registered Dietitians in the Health Care System." *Acad Nutr Diet J* 111 (2011): 813–815.
15. Haughton, B., and J. Stang. "Population Risk Factors and Trends in Health Care and Public Policy." *Acad Nutr Diet J* 112 (2012): S35–S46.
16. See Note 9.

17. Quagliane, D., M. Hermann. "Communicating Accurate Food and Nutrition Information." Practice Paper of the Academy of Nutrition and Dietetics. *Acad Nutr Diet J* 2012 (112): 759.

18. American Dietetic Association. "Position of the American Dietetic Association: Food and Nutrition Misinformation." *J Am Diet Assoc* 106 (2006): 601–606.

19. Rowe, S., and N. Alexander. "Communicating Dietary Guidelines to a Balking Public." *Nutr Today* 44, no. 2 (2009): 81–84.

20. Ayres, E.J. "2011 Nutrition Informatics." *Acad Nutr Diet J* 112 (2012): 350–367.

21. See Note 20.

22. Academy of Nutrition and Dietetics. "Top Three Dynamic Initiatives for Practice and Education." Accessed June 1, 2012, www.eatright.org

23. Merrifield, R., J. Calhoun, and D. Steven. "The Next Revolution in Productivity." *Harvard Business Review* (June 2008): 2–9.

24. Ayyagari, R. "Technostress Antecedents and Implications." *MIS Quarterly* 35 (2011): 831–858.

25. Cappellano, K.L. "Living Green." *Nutr Today* 44 (2009): 38–42.

26. Harmon, A.H., B.L. Gerald, and ADA. "Position Paper: Position of the American Dietetic Association: Food and Nutrition Professionals Can Implement Practices to Conserve Natural Resources and Support Ecological Sustainability." *J Am Diet Assoc* 107 (2007): 1033–1043.

27. Mills, L.S. "From Local Chow to Green Machines; ADA Members Are Turning Foodservice into Eco-Friendly Operations." *ADA Times* (January–February 2008): 12–16.

28. Arose, S. "A Guide to Greener Meetings." *J Am Diet Assoc* 109 (2009): 800–802.

29. Camp, K., and F.J. Rohr. "Advanced Practitioners and What They Do That Is Different: Roles in Genetics." *Top Clin Nutr* 24, no. 3 (2009): 219–230.

30. DeBusk, R.M., C.P. Fogarty, J.M. Ordovas, and K.S. Kornman. "Nutritional Genomics in Practice. Where Do We Begin?" *J Am Diet Assoc* 105 (2005): 589–598.

31. De Busk, R. "Diet-Related Disease. Nutritional Genomics, and Food and Nutrition Professionals." *J Am Diet Assoc* 109 (2009): 410–413.

32. Trujillo, E.,C. Davis, and J. Milner. "Nutrigenomics, Proteomics, Metabolomics, and the Practice of Dietetics." *J Am Diet Assoc* 106 (2006): 403–413.

33. Weston, A.D., and L. Hood. "Systems Biology, Proteomics, and the Future of Healthcare: Toward Predictive, Preventative, and Personalized Medicine." *J Proteome Res* 3, no. 2 (2004): 179–196.

34. German, J.B., S.M. Watkins, and L.Fay. "Metabolomics in Practice: Emerging Knowledge to Guide Future Dietetic Advice Toward Individualized Health." *J AmDiet Assoc* 105 (2005): 1425–1432.

35. Reilly, P.R, and R.M. DeBusk. "Ethical and Legal Issues in Nutritional Genomics." *J Am Diet Assoc* 108(2008): 36–40.

36. Kauwell, G.P. "Epigenetics: What It Is and How It Can Affect Dietetics Practice." *J Am Diet Assoc* 108 (2008): 1056–1059.

37. Srump, P.J., R. Weiss, J.W. Newman, J.A. Pennington, K.L. Tucker, P.L. Wisenfeld, A.K. Illner, D.M.L. Kurfeld, and J. Kaput. "Web Enabled and Improved Software Tools and Data Are Needed to Measure Nutrient Intakes and Physical Activity for Personalized Health Research." *J Nutr* 140 (2010): 2104–2115.

38. Institute of Medicine. Food and Nutrition Board. *Dietary Reference Intakes: The Essential Guide to Nutrient Requirements.* (Washington, DC: National Academies Press, 2006).

39. U.S. Food and Drug Administration. "Fact Sheet: FDA Nanotechnology Task Force Report Outlines, Scientific, Regulatory Challenges." National Nanotechnology Initiative, Accessed July 11, 2012, www.nano.gov

40. Nickols-Richardson, S.M. "Nanotechnology: Implications for Food and Nutrition Professionals." *J Am Diet Assoc* 107 (2007): 1494–1497.

41. Srinivas, P.R., M. Philbert, T.Q. Vu, Q. Huang, J.L. Kokini, E. Saltos, H. Chen, et al. "Nanotechnology Research: Applications in Nutritional Sciences." *J Nutr* 140 (2010): 119–124.

42. Rosen, R., C. Earthman, I. Marquart, and M. Reicka. "Continuing Education Needs of Registered Dietitians Regarding Nutrigemomics." *J Amer Diet Assoc* 106 (2006): 1242–1245.

43. Jeffries, D., M. Johnson, and J. Ravens. "Nurturing and Nourishing: The Nurse's Role in Nutritional Care." *J Clin Nurs* 20 (2011): 317–330.

44. Bland, J. "The Future of Nutritional Pharmacology." *Altern Ther* 14 (2008): 12–14.

45. House of Delegates Report. "Key Trends Affecting the Dietetics Profession and the American Dietetic Association." *J Am Diet Assoc* 102 (2002): S1821–S1939.

46. "President's Page: At the Tipping Point: Changing Our World." *Acad Nutr Diet J.* 112 (2012): 16.

47. Maletz, F.W. "From Hospital to 'Healthspital.'" *Futurist.* (March–April 2011): p. 17–19.

48. Lafferty, L. Personal communication, July 7, 2012.

49. Academy of Nutrition and Dietetics. "Projections and Opportunities for an Increasing Demand for Dietetics Practitioners: 2011 Dietetics Workforce Demand Study Results and Recommendations." *J Acad Nutr Diet J* 112, Suppl. (2012): 1.

50. Peregrin, J. "Next on the Menu: Labeling Law Could Mean New Career Opportunities for RDs." *J Am Diet Assoc* 110 (2011): S12–S14.

51. "Position of the American Dietetic Association: Functional Foods." *J Am Diet Assoc* 1090 (2009): 735–746.

52. Institute of Medicine. *Dietary Reference Intakes.* Washington D.C: National Academies Press, 2012 Preface, p. viii.

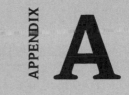

Code of Ethics for the Profession of Dietetics and Process for Consideration of Ethics Issues (2009)

PREAMBLE

The American Dietetic Association (ADA) and its credentialing agency, the Commission on Dietetic Registration (CDR), believe it is in the best interest of the profession and the public it serves to have a Code of Ethics in place that provides guidance to dietetic practitioners in their professional practice and conduct. Dietetics practitioners have voluntarily adopted this Code of Ethics to reflect the values and ethical principles guiding the dietetics profession and to set forth commitments and obligations of the dietetics practitioner to the public, clients, the profession, colleagues, and other professionals. The current Code of Ethics was approved on June 2, 2009, by the ADA Board of Directors, House of Delegates, and the Commission on Dietetic Registration.

APPLICATION

The Code of Ethics applies to the following practitioners:

(a) In its entirety to members of ADA who are Registered Dietitians or Dietetic Technicians.

(b) Except for sections dealing solely with the credential, to all members of ADA who are not RDs or DTRs; and

(c) Except for aspects dealing solely with membership, to all RDs and DTRs who are not members of ADA.

FUNDAMENTAL PRINCIPLES

1. The dietetics practitioner conducts himself/herself with honesty, integrity, and fairness.

2. The dietetics practitioner supports and promotes high standards of professional practice. The dietetics practitioner accepts the obligation to protect clients, the public, and the profession by upholding the Code of Ethics for the profession of Dietetics and by reporting perceived violations of the Code through the processes established by ADA and its credentialing agency, CDR.

3. The dietetics practitioner considers the health, safety, and welfare of the public at all times.

4. The dietetics practitioner complies with all laws and regulations applicable or related to the profession or to the practitioner's ethical obligations as described in this Code.

5. The dietetics practitioner provides professional services with objectivity and with respect for the unique needs and values of individuals.

6. The dietetics practitioner does not engage in false or misleading practices or communications.

7. The dietetics practitioner withdraws from professional practice when unable to fulfill his or her professional duties and responsibilities to clients and others.

8. The dietetics practitioner recognizes and exercises professional judgment within the limits of his or her qualifications and collaborates with others, seeks counsel, or makes referrals as appropriate.

9. The dietetics practitioner treats clients and patients with respect and consideration.

10. The dietetics practitioner protects confidential information and makes full disclosure about any limitations on his or her ability to guarantee full confidentiality.
11. The dietetics practitioner, in dealing with and providing services to clients and others, complies with the same principles set forth above.
12. The dietetics practitioner practices dietetics based on evidence-based principles and current information.
13. The dietetics practitioner presents reliable and substantiated information and interprets controversial information without personal bias, recognizing that legitimate differences of opinion exist.
14. The dietetics practitioner assumes a life-long responsibility and accountability for personal competence in practice, consistent with accepted professional standards, continually striving to increase professional knowledge and skills and to apply them in practice.
15. The dietetics practitioner is alert to the occurrence of a real or potential conflict of interest and takes appropriate action whenever a conflict arises.
16. The dietetics practitioner permits the use of his or her name for the purpose of certifying that dietetics services have been rendered only if he or she has provided or supervised the provision of those services.
17. The dietetics practitioner accurately presents professional qualifications and credentials.
18. The dietetics practitioner does not invite, accept, or offer gifts, monetary incentives, or other considerations that affect or reasonably give an appearance of affecting his/her professional judgment.
19. The dietetics practitioner demonstrates respect for the values, rights, knowledge, and skills of colleagues and other professionals.

Bylaws of the Academy of Nutrition and Dietetics—Article II

MEMBERS

Section 1. Classes of Members. The Academy shall have the following five (5) classes of members:

Active   Retired   Student   Honorary   International

Section 2. Active Members Qualifications.

2a. An individual holding a baccalaureate degree from a regionally accredited college or university, and meeting the academic requirement specified by the Academy, plus one or more of the following criteria may apply for Active membership: a Registered Dietitian ("RD") credentialed by the Commission on Dietetic Registration ("CDR"); completed an academic and/or supervised practice program accredited by the Accreditation Council for Education in Nutrition and Dietetics ("ACEND").

2b. An individual holding a master's or a doctoral degree, and a degree (baccalaureate, master's, doctoral) in one of the following areas may apply for Active membership: dietetics, foods, and nutrition, nutrition, community/public health nutrition, food science, or food service systems management. A regionally accredited college or university must have conferred each degree.

2c. An individual meeting one or more of the following criteria may apply for Active membership: a Dietetic Technician, Registered ("DTR") credentialed by the CDR or has established eligibility to take the examination for dietetic technicians; completed an ACEND approved associate degree program for dietetic technicians; holds a baccalaureate degree and meets the academic requirements specified by ACEND, and has completed an ACEND accredited/approved dietetic technician program experience.

2d. An individual who previously paid the optional one-time dues in order to obtain "life" membership in the Academy, or has completed a term as President of the Academy.

Section 3. Retired Members Qualifications. Any dietetics professional qualifying for the Active membership category that is no longer employed in dietetic practice or education and is at least sixty-two (62) years of age, or is retired on total (permanent) disability may apply for Retired membership.

Section 4. Student Members Qualifications. Student classification can be held for a maximum of six (6) years. An individual meeting one of the following criteria may apply for Student membership:

4a. A student enrolled in an ACEND accredited/approved program;

4b. A student in a regionally accredited college or university who state his/her intent to enter an ACEND accredited/approved program;

4c. Active members returning to school on a full-time basis for a baccalaureate or graduate degree in a dietetic related course of study may apply for Student membership status.

Section 5. Honorary Members Qualifications. An individual who has made a notable contribution to the field of nutrition and dietetics may be admitted to the Academy as an Honorary member upon invitation of the Board of Directors.

Section 6. International Members Qualifications. An individual who has completed formal training in food, nutrition or dietetics outside the United States and U.S. Territories verified by the country's professional dietetics association and/or country's regulatory body.

Section 7. Privileges of Membership.

7a. Active Members. Active members whose dues are not in arrears shall be entitled one vote in each matter submitted to vote of members and are eligible to hold elected and appointed offices and positions at the national level. Active members shall be eligible to hold elected and appointed offices and positions at the affiliate level as designated by the affiliate dietetic association.

7b. Retired Members. Retired members whose dues are not in arrears shall be entitled to all the rights of the Active membership category.

7c. Student Members. Student members whose dues are not in arrears shall have the right to vote in the national and affiliate elections and are eligible to hold appointed positions at the national and affiliate levels if a resident of the United States or U.S. Territories. Student members shall not have a right to hold elected positions on the national and affiliate levels.

7d. Honorary Members. Honorary members may serve as members of committees and attend meetings. Honorary members shall not be entitled to vote and eligible to hold elected office.

7e. International Members. International members may be members of committees and attend meetings. International members shall be entitled to vote and eligible to hold elected office at the affiliate level.

7f. Voting. Each member eligible to vote shall be entitled to one vote on each matter submitted to a vote of the members.

Section 8. Termination and Reinstatement of Membership. The Board of Directors or its designee may terminate a member in default in the payment of dues. The House of Delegates ("HOD") or its disignee may terminate membership for cause. Any former member who forfeited membership for nonpayment of dues may be reinstated to their former classification by paying the current annual dues and a reinstatement fee, and meeting the Academy's reinstatement requirements. Former members from the retired and returning student classes will be reinstated into the active class. Any former member whose membership was terminated for cause may request reinstatement of membership following one (1) year of termination unless otherwise determined by the HOD.

Source: Reproduced with permission of Academy of Nutrition and Dietetics. "Bylaws of the Academy of Nutrition and Dietetics - Article II" 2012.

Associate Members

Academy of Nutrition and Dietetics Associates are required to hold a minimum of a baccalaureate degree granted by a U.S. regionally accredited college or university or foreign equivalent. The appropriate degree and training, certification, or license in one of the following food/culinary and health-related professions meets the qualifications for an Academy Associate.

- Certified Health Education Specialist (CHES)
- Certified Midwife (CN or CNM)
- Certified Professional, Food Safety (CP-FS)*
- Dental Hygienist (BS-DH or RDH or LDH)
- Dentist (DDS)
- Pharmacist (RPH or PharmD)
- Physical or Occupational Therapist (PT/OT)
- Physician (ND or DO)
- Physician Assistant (PA)
- Registered Environmental Health
- Specialist/Registered Sanitation (REHS/RS)
- Registered Nurse (RN)*
- School Nutrition Specialist (SNS)*
- Speech-Language Pathologist (CCC-SLP)

- Degree in Culinary Arts from a U.S. regionally accredited college or university or U.S. culinary association*
- Certification from the American Culinary Foundation or the International Association of Culinary Professionals*
- Certification from the American College of Sports Medicine*
- Certification from the Dietary Managers Association*

*Proof of Bachelor's degree required
Source: www.eatright.org. (Accessed June 22, 2011). Reprinted by permission of Academy of Nutrition and Dietetics.

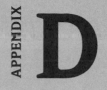

Academy of Nutrition and Dietetics Organization Charts

Academy of Nutrition and Dietetics Organization Charts

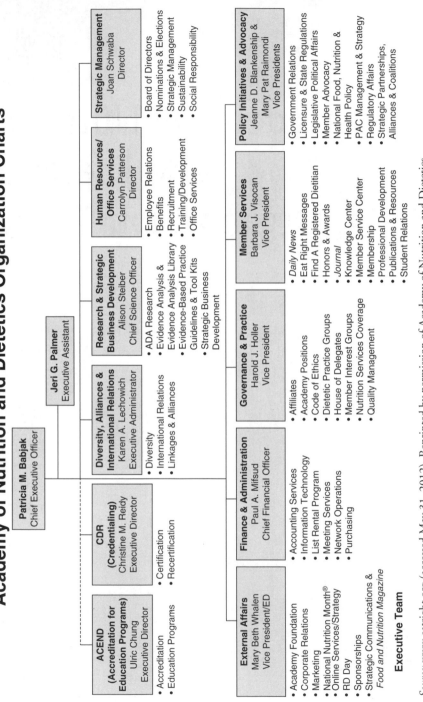

Patricia M. Babjak
Chief Executive Officer

Jeri G. Palmer
Executive Assistant

ACEND (Accreditation for Education Programs)
Ulric Chung
Executive Director
- Accreditation
- Education Programs

CDR (Credentialing)
Christine M. Reidy
Executive Director
- Certification
- Recertification

Diversity, Alliances & International Relations
Karen A. Lechowich
Executive Administrator
- Diversity
- International Relations
- Linkages & Alliances

Research & Strategic Business Development
Alison Steiber
Chief Science Officer
- ADA Research
- Evidence Analysis &
- Evidence Analysis Library
- Evidence-Based Practice Guidelines & Tool Kits
- Strategic Business Development

Human Resources/ Office Services
Carrolyn Patterson
Director
- Employee Relations
- Benefits
- Recruitment
- Training/Development
- Office Services

Strategic Management
Joan Schwaba
Director
- Board of Directors
- Nominations & Elections
- Strategic Management
- Sustainability
- Social Responsibility

External Affairs
Mary Beth Whalen
Vice President/ED
- Academy Foundation
- Corporate Relations
- Marketing
- National Nutrition Month®
- Online Services/Strategy
- RD Day
- Sponsorships
- Strategic Communications &
Food and Nutrition Magazine

Finance & Administration
Paul A. Mifsud
Chief Financial Officer
- Accounting Services
- Information Technology
- List Rental Program
- Meeting Services
- Network Operations
- Purchasing

Governance & Practice
Harold J. Holler
Vice President
- Affiliates
- Academy Positions
- Code of Ethics
- Dietetic Practice Groups
- House of Delegates
- Member Interest Groups
- Nutrition Services Coverage
- Quality Management

Member Services
Barbara J. Visocan
Vice President
- *Daily News*
- Eat Right Messages
- Find A Registered Dietitian
- Honors & Awards
- *Journal*
- Knowledge Center
- Member Service Center
- Membership
- Professional Development
- Publications & Resources
- Student Relations

Policy Initiatives & Advocacy
Jeanne D. Blankenship &
Mary Pat Raimondi
Vice Presidents
- Government Relations
- Licensure & State Regulations
- Legislative Political Affairs
- Member Advocacy
- National Food, Nutrition & Health Policy
- PAC Management & Strategy
- Regulatory Affairs
- Strategic Partnerships, Alliances & Coalitions

Executive Team

Source: www.eatright.org (accessed May 31, 2012). Reprinted by permission of Academy of Nutrition and Dietetics.

Sub-Units of Dietetic Practice Groups and Member Interest Groups

DIETETIC PRACTICE GROUP SUB-UNITS

A Dietetic Practice Group (DPG) may develop recognized sub-units or groups of members within the DPG based on a practice area or issue of interest to the members of the DPG. Currently over 30 of these sub-specialty areas exist within the main DPGs. The current list is as follows:

Name of Sub-Unit	DPG Affiliation
Food and Nutrition Informatics	CNM
Home Care	DHCC
Corrections	DHCC
Food Safety	FCP
Restaurant and Retail Food Service	FCP
Supermarket	FCP
Commercial and Retail Food Service	MFNS
Dietitians in Gluten Intolerance Disease	MNPG

(continues)

Name of Sub-Unit	DPG Affiliation
Dietitians in Physical Medicine and Rehabilitation	MNPG
Authors	NE
Private Practice	NE
Corporate Health	NE
Technology and Social Media	NE
Speakers	NE
Health Coaches	NE
Marketing and Public Relations	NE
Children with Special Health Care Needs	PNPG
Infant Nutrition/Breastfeeding with Neonatology	PNPG
Diabetes, Wellness and Weight Management	PNPG
Failure to Thrive, Gastroenterology and Allergy	PNPG
Nutrition Support Services	PNPG
Eating Disorder/Adolescents	PNPG
Clinical and Translational Science	RDPG
Disordered Eating and Eating Disorders (DEED)	SCAN
Wellness/CV	SCAN
Sports Dietetics USA	SCAN
Bariatrics	WM
Padiatric Weight Management	WM

MEMBER INTEREST GROUPS (MIGs)

Member interest groups (MIGs) focus on areas other than the practice of dietetics or geographic location in current groups.

Chinese Americans in Dietetics and Nutrition (CADN)
CADN members serve, educate, promote research, and share work experience with the community to enhance the nutritional status of the Chinese in the United States.

Fifty Plus in Nutrition and Dietetics (FPIND)
FPIND focuses on programming education, careers, and networking target audiences.

Filipino Americans in Dietetics and Nutrition (FADAN)
FADAN fosters networking, mentoring, and support for professional issues diverse culture and ethnicity of this population.

Jewish Member Interest Group (JMIG)
JMIG provides credible resources regarding cultural competencies concerning kosher in observance of kashrut (dietary law) meal service customs to their clients.

Latinos and Hispanics in Dietetics and Nutrition (LAHIDAN)
LAHIDAN fosters the development and improvement of food, nutrition, and States and related territories.

Muslims in Dietetics and Nutrition (MIDAN)
MIDAN serves members with an interest in cross-cultural awareness and to the Muslim population. This may include those who are of the Muslim faith.

National Organization of Blacks in Dietetics and Nutrition (NOBIDAN)
NOBIDAN provides a forum for professional development of food and nutrition, optimal nutrition, and well-being for the general public, particularly those of African descent.

National Organization of Men in Nutrition (NOMIN)
NOMIN promotes careers in food and nutrition and professional growth of dissemination of information regarding men's health issues.

Thirty and Under in Nutrition and Dietetics (TUND)
TUND empowers young practitioners to network and collaborate as the nation's future food and nutrition leaders.

Source: Reprinted by permission of Academy of Nutrition and Dietetics.

Position Paper Update 2012

The House of Delegates (HOD) approved the proposed position paper concept "The Role of Nutrition Genomics in Dietetics" in January 2011. The position paper is under development. Publication is planned for early 2013. The following is a list of all current positions of the Academy of Nutrition and Dietetics.

FOOD CHOICES

- Total diet approach to communicating food and nutrition information. *J Am Diet Assoc.* 2007;107(7):1224–1232. (Reaffirmed, update to be published in 2012)
- Vegetarian diets. *J Am Diet Assoc.* 2009;109(7):1266–1282. (Expires 2013)
- Health implications of dietary fiber. *J Am Diet Assoc.* 2008;108(10): 1716–1731. (Expires 2013)
- Functional foods. *J Am Diet Assoc.* 2009;109(4):735–746. (Reaffirmed, update to be published in 2012)
- Dietary fatty acids. *J Am Diet Assoc.* 2007;107(9):1599–1611. (Reaffirmed, update to be published in 2012)

FOOD SUPPLY

- **Safety**
  Food and water safety. *J Am Diet Assoc.* 2009;109(8):1449–1460.
  (Reaffirmed, update to be published in 2012)
- **Supplementation/Fortification**
  The impact of fluoride on health. *J Am Diet Assoc.* 2005;105(8):
  1620–1628. (Reaffirmed, update to be published in 2012)
  Nutrient supplementation. *J Am Diet Assoc.* 2009;109(12):
  2073–2085. (Expires 2013)
- **Substitutes**
  Use of nutritive and nonnutritive sweeteners. *J Am Diet Assoc.*
  2004;104(2):225–275. (Reaffirmed, update to be published in
  2012)
- **Food Security/Environment**
  Agricultural and food biotechnology. *J Am Diet Assoc.* 2006;106(2):
  285–293. (Reaffirmed, update to be published in 2012)
  Food insecurity in the US. *J Am Diet Assoc.* 2010;110(9):1368–1376.
  (Expires 2014)
  Addressing world hunger, malnutrition, and food insecurity. *J Am
  Diet Assoc.* 2003;103(8):1046–1057. (Reaffirmed, update to be
  published in 2012)

LIFE SPAN

- **Pregnancy/Breastfeeding**
  Promoting and supporting breastfeeding. *J Am Diet Assoc.*
  2009;109(11):1926–1942. (Expires 2013)
  Nutrition and lifestyle for a healthy pregnancy outcome. *J Am Diet
  Assoc.* 2008;108(3):553–561. (Reaffirmed, update and new prac-
  tice paper on the same topic to be published in 2012)
  Obesity, reproduction, and pregnancy outcomes. *J Am Diet Assoc.*
  2009;109(5):918–927. Academy, American Society for Nutrition
  Joint Position. (Reaffirmed, update to be published in 2012)
- **Infancy/Childhood**
  Child and adolescent nutrition assistance programs. *J Am Diet Assoc.*
  2010;110(5):791–799. (Expires 2014)

Nutrition guidance for healthy children ages 2–11 years. *J Am Diet Assoc.* 2008;108(7):1038–1047. (Reaffirmed, update to be published in 2012)

Local support for nutrition integrity in schools. *J Am Diet Assoc.* 2010;110(7):1244–1254. (Expires 2014)

Benchmarks for nutrition in child care. *J Am Diet Assoc.* 2011;111(4):607–615. (Expires 2015)

Comprehensive school nutrition services. *J Am Diet Assoc.* 2010;110(11):1738–1749. Academy, School Nutrition Association and Society for Nutrition Education Joint Position. (Expires 2014)

- **Adults**

Nutrition and athletic performance for adults. *J Am Diet Assoc.* 2009;109(3):509–527. Academy, Dietitians of Canada and American College of Sports Medicine Joint Position. (Expires 2012)

- **Older Adults**

Individualized nutrition approaches for older adults in health care communities. *J Am Diet Assoc.* 2010;110(10):1549–1553. (Expires 2014)

Nutrition across the spectrum of aging. *J Am Diet Assoc.* 2005; 105(4):616–633. (Reaffirmed, update to be published in 2012)

Food and nutrition programs for community-residing older adults. *J Am Diet Assoc.* 2010;110(3):463–472. Academy, American Society for Nutrition and Society for Nutrition Education Joint Position. (Expires 2014)

NUTRITION MANAGEMENT

- **Disease/Special Conditions**

Nutrition intervention in the treatment eating disorders. *J Am Diet Assoc.* 2011;111(8):1236–1241. (Expires 2014)

Nutrition intervention and human immunodeficiency virus infection. *J Am Diet Assoc.* 2010;110(7):1105–1119. (Expires 2014)

Providing nutrition services for people with development disabilities and special health care needs. *J Am Diet Assoc.* 2010;110(2): 296–307. (Expires 2013)

Ethical and legal issues in nutrition, hydration, and feeding. *J Am Diet Assoc.* 2008;108(5):873–882. (Reaffirmed, update and new practice paper on the same topic to be published in 2012)
- **MNT/Health Care**
  Integration of medical nutrition therapy and pharmacotherapy. *J Am Diet Assoc.* 2010;110(6):950–956. (Expires 2014)
- **Weight Management**
  Weight management. *J Am Diet Assoc.* 2009;109(2):330–346. (Expires 2013)
  Individual-, family-, school-, and community-based interventions for pediatric overweight. *J Am Diet Assoc.* 2006;106(6):925–945. (Reaffirmed, update to be published in 2012)

PUBLIC HEALTH

- Oral health and nutrition. *J Am Diet Assoc.* 2007;107(8):1418–1428. (Reaffirmed, update and new practice paper on the same topic to be published in 2012)
- The roles of registered dietitians and dietetic technicians, registered in health promotion and disease prevention. *J Am Diet Assoc.* 2006;106(11):1875–1884. (Reaffirmed, update and new practice paper on the same topic to be published in 2012)

ACCESSING ACADEMY POSITIONS

- Positions are available for viewing from the Academy website at: http://www.eatright.org/positions/. PDF copies may be downloaded from the website. Single copies of positions can be mailed or faxed upon request by contacting Academy Headquarters (800/877-1600, ext. 4892 or e-mail ppapers@eatright.org).

CONTACT

- Donna L. Wickstrom, MS, RD, at Academy Headquarters (800/877-1600, ext. 4835 or e-mail, ppapers@eatright.org) for answers to your questions on Academy positions.

Source: © 2012 Academy of Nutrition and Dietetics. Reprinted by permission of Academy of Nutrition and Dietetics.

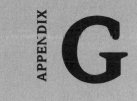
Dietetics Career
Development Guide

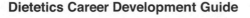

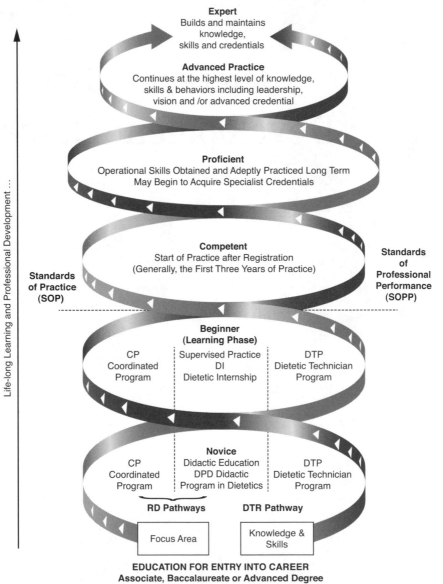

Dietetics Career Development Guide

Expert
Builds and maintains knowledge, skills and credentials

Advanced Practice
Continues at the highest level of knowledge, skills & behaviors including leadership, vision and /or advanced credential

Proficient
Operational Skills Obtained and Adeptly Practiced Long Term
May Begin to Acquire Specialist Credentials

Competent
Start of Practice after Registration
(Generally, the First Three Years of Practice)

Standards of Practice (SOP)

Standards of Professional Performance (SOPP)

Beginner (Learning Phase)

| CP Coordinated Program | Supervised Practice DI Dietetic Internship | DTP Dietetic Technician Program |

Novice

| CP Coordinated Program | Didactic Education DPD Didactic Program in Dietetics | DTP Dietetic Technician Program |

RD Pathways   **DTR Pathway**

Focus Area   Knowledge & Skills

EDUCATION FOR ENTRY INTO CAREER
Associate, Baccalaureate or Advanced Degree

Life-long Learning and Professional Development ...

Definition of Dietetics: Dietetics is the integration, application and communication of principles derived from food, nutrition, social, business and basic sciences, to achieve and maintain optimal nutrition status of individuals through the development, provision and management of effective food and nutrition services in a variety of settings.

Source: © Academy of Nutrition and Dietetics. Reprinted by permission of Academy of Nutrition and Dietetics.

Index

Figures and tables are indicated by *f* and *t* following the page number.